CM Francis

Medical Ethics

CM Francis

Medical Ethics

As per revised MCI curriculum

Fourth Edition

Revised and Edited by

Rimpi Gupta MBBS MS (Anatomy)
Assistant Professor
Department of Anatomy
Kalpana Chawla Government Medical College (KCGMC)
Karnal, Haryana, India

JAYPEE BROTHERS MEDICAL PUBLISHERS
The Health Sciences Publisher
New Delhi | London

Jaypee Brothers Medical Publishers (P) Ltd

Headquarters
EMCA House, 23/23-B
Ansari Road, Daryaganj
New Delhi 110 002, India
Landline: +91-11-23272143, +91-11-23272703
+91-11-23282021, +91-11-23245672
e-mail: jaypee@jaypeebrothers.com

Corporate Office
4838/24, Ansari Road, Daryaganj
New Delhi 110 002, India
Phone: +91-11-43574357
Fax: +91-11-43574314
e-mail: jaypee@jaypeebrothers.com

Overseas Office
JP Medical Ltd.
83, Victoria Street, London
SW1H 0HW (UK)
Phone: +44-20 3170 8910
e-mail: info@jpmedpub.com

EU GPSR Authorised Representative
Logos Europe, 9 rue Nicolas Poussin
17000, La Rochelle, France
Phone: +33 (0) 6 67 93 73 78
e-mail: contact@logoseurope.eu

Website: www.jaypeebrothers.com

Website: www.jaypeedigital.com

Medical Ethics

First Edition	:	1993
Second Edition	:	2004
Third Edition	:	2017
Fourth Edition	:	**2020**
Reprint	:	**2026**

ISBN 978-93-89188-62-2

Printed at: Samrat Offset Pvt. Ltd.

Preface to the Fourth Edition

The third edition of *Medical Ethics* has gained a warm response by the health professionals and others. It enabled them to reflect on the various ethical issues encountered by them in daily clinical practice and to find appropriate solutions. The book has been recommended by various Universities of Health Sciences in India and abroad.

In the era of technology, every person is well aware of his rights to health care, so a health professional should be able to understand the concept of medical ethics, professionalism including language and communication skills, leadership quality and computer skills apart from core medical education.

It has become a common practice by public to target health professionals which also includes violence against doctors. One such incidence happened recently in the state of West Bengal which became a national issue. Also, the #MeToo movement was critical in giving voice to the victims of sexual misconduct leading to health professionals being sensitive to gender neutral interpersonal communication with efforts made to nurture the craft of professional behavior.

From the current session, the Medical Council of India (MCI) has introduced new medical curriculum which includes foundation course of one month duration at the entry level of a student to a medical college. MCI has laid emphasis on "AETCOM" (Attitude, Ethics, Communication) module which is a welcome step.

An increasing awareness of the need for understanding the ethical issues encountered by the health professionals all over the world has brought the teaching/learning of medical and bioethics as an integral and essential part of medical curriculum. The book has been revised according to new MCI curriculum with the hope that the book will be useful in the teaching/learning of *Medical Ethics* and it will address the issues of health care in modern world.

All the chapters have been updated and expanded. The new edition of the book includes the recent guidelines by MCI enabling health-care professionals to serve their patients and the society in a better way.

Rimpi Gupta

Preface to the First Edition

The question of medical ethics has been raised at numerous meetings and conferences of medical professionals and others. There is a general feeling that not enough attention is being paid to this important question and there are not enough guidelines for the professionals to follow, especially in the fast changing situation.

Recently, I was invited to participate in an international seminar on "Transcultural dimensions in medical and bioethics". The deliberations at the seminar brought to the fore differences in the perceptions of ethical problems by people in different cultures. With better and quicker communication, and doctors trained in one culture practising in another, there are bound to be situations where conflicts in thinking and approach to medical and bioethics could take place.

The health professional faces ethical problems everywhere and all the time. Choices have to be made in consonance with the value systems held by the society and the profession in the particular cultural milieu. Newer issues come up all the time. Changes are fast and the doctor has to make decisions, even though there may not be sufficient guidelines.

The newer issues may be in diverse fields—advances in technology, genetics or diseases like AIDS. Reproductive technologies produce ethical issues of a magnitude not known earlier. There are ethical issues involved in the right to health, health policies and distributive justice in health care.

It is necessary for every doctor to be aware of the existing problems. The doctor should also be trained to analyze newer problems as they arise and deal with them in a acceptable manner keeping in view the socioeconomic-cultural situation in which he is practising. Unfortunately the standard of training in medical and bioethics today leaves much to be desired. Very few medical colleges have medical ethics as a subject of learning/teaching. There are some basic topics dealt under forensic medicine which really do not help when the doctor enters the field of medical practice, whether private or institution-based.

This book is written with the hope that the doctors in the country are enabled to solve issues in ethics in the medical and health care of the people with less tension and more understanding.

CM Francis

Contents

SECTION 7

EMERGING ISSUES

SECTION 8

HUMAN EXPERIMENTATION AND RESEARCH

CHAPTER 1

Medical Ethics: Some Basic Issues

Ethics deals with the right conduct. It helps in the distinction between what is considered right or wrong at a given time, in a given culture, with the moral consequences of the action. We face different choices of conduct. Often, none of the alternatives appears to be entirely satisfactory. Situations of ambiguity and uncertainty have to be faced and in dilemmas we have to make our specific choice.

WHICH WAY TO GO?

Ethics is derived from *ethos*. There are distinctive attitudes pervading the culture of a group of persons, with adherence to certain values. It includes a definite tradition, and sharing in customs and experiences. There is now a tension between traditional ethics and the changing values and insights. Contemporary ethos strives to preserve what is essential in the older traditions and modifies others according to changes in the perception of the society. It varies from one culture to another.

Is there a transcultural ethics? There are certain values which are common to humanity. Hence, there can be some commonality in ethics. People are coming together more easily now. The interaction and exchange of views influence the thinking of each other and also helps in forming some common shared ethics. However, there will be differences in the detailed perceptions of what is ethical and what is moral between various cultures.

Every profession has an *ethical* code. It fosters and guarantees the ethos. It assures the members of the profession and the public a standard of professional relationships. The ethical code makes the ethos more concrete. The code verbalises the ethos. It defines the norms. Ethical code is different from legislation. Often it does away with the need for legislation. The code serves as a guide. All members of the profession are expected to adhere to the code.

There is need for ethical or righteous conduct in all our endeavours.

"Sukarthah Sarvabutanam
Matah sarvah pravarthayah
Sukham ca na vina dharmat
Thasmad dharmaparo bhavet"
—Vagbhata in *Astanga Hridaya*

(All activities of man are directed to the end of attaining happiness, whereas happiness is never achieved without righteousness. It is the bounden duty of man to be righteous in his action)

Medical ethics is a part of general ethics. It is the application of what is good and right derived from values in health care. It deals with those norms that govern the behavior of the medical profession. It is concerned with the obligations of the doctor to the patient, other doctors and health professionals and the society. Medical ethics is a systematic effort to work within the ethos of medicine, which has traditionally been service to the sick.

"In all circumstances and to the best of your ability, strive to alleviate the suffering of the patient and heal him/her".

There is now a shift from the traditional individual patient doctor relationship of medical care. With the changes in knowledge and skills and the needs of the patients, their families and the community, there is an increased concern with the health of the society in general. There is a shift to greater accountability to the society and more comprehensive health care.

Doctors and other health professionals are confronted with issues other than technical ones. Our relationships with patients and people bring about many sociological problems, superimposed on the strictly medical or health problems. With the advances in science and technology, these problems are on the increase. The great successes in technological advance, treatment and management during the past few decades have themselves brought up a host of problems.

> *"The world that we have made as a result of the level of thinking we have done so far, creates problems we cannot solve at the level we created them".*
>
> —Albert Einstein

India has a hoary past in medicine. There was emphasis on ethics in general and ethics in medical practice in particular. *Dharma* (ethical conduct according to one's state) has been a very important concept in Indian culture and thought.

VALUES IN MEDICINE

The ethical conduct arises from many values, the most important being the concept of love for the neighbor. This is seen in most scriptures. Love for the neighbor is one of the two important tenets of the Christian religion. "You must love your neighbour as yourself". In India, the *Vedas* explained why one should love the neighbour. Love your neighbor because your neighbor is in truth your very self and what separates you from him (her) is illusion (*maya*) and each one of us has in us *atman*, a part of *paramatman*. *Charaka Samhita* (6th century BC) states: "He who practises not for money nor for caprice but out of compassion for living beings (*Bhuta-daya*) is the best among all physicians. Hard is it to find a conferer of religious blessings comparable to the physician who snaps the snares of death for his patients. The physician who regards compassion for living beings as the highest religion fulfills his mission (*siddarthah*) and obtains the highest happiness".

Very high value is placed on human life. There is, therefore, respect for life, irrespective of age, nationality, sex, color, religion or social status. There is also high value placed on the quality of life.

Medicine presupposes certain fundamental values:
- preservation of life,
- relief of suffering,
- cure of disease,
- care of the person,
- prevention of disease, and
- promotion of health.

Based on these and other values, the doctor has certain obligations. There is need for fidelity to the interests of the patient.

There must exist *trust*. It follows that there must be confidentiality and truth-telling. But difficulties crop up when you weigh obligation to tell the truth versus obligation to protect the well-being of the patient. There can be fear in the mind of the doctor; will my honest description of the condition upset the patient seriously and even affect recovery?

There will be conflicts when applying the values. When there is conflict between two values, which value will take precedence? The rights and freedom of the individual may conflict with the needs of the society. One issue will be the use of personal information. The individual values privacy. There can be conflict between fidelity to the patient's and the physician's personal interests (financial and others).

Medicine as a Profession

There are serious criticisms of the medical profession today: its lack of accountability, its structure and organization, its dependence on technology and its failure to address important issues in health.

There are two roles for the doctor: Physician-healer and **physician-professional**. The two are linked together; the doctor must function effectively in both the roles. The **healer** offers advice and support in matters of health and ministers to the sick. Later, **professionalism** was developed; it joined the tradition of the healer as a means of organising and supporting the services to the people. Laws governing licensure and registration gave the profession a broad monopoly over health care.

WHAT IS A PROFESSION?

A profession is defined as an occupation which "one professes to be skilled in and to follow:

a. A vocation in which a professed knowledge of a department of learning or science is used in its application to the affairs of others or in the practice of an art founded on it;
b. In a wider sense; any calling or occupation by which a person habitually earns his living"

—*Oxford English Dictionary*

The definition includes:

- 'Profession': Its ancient meaning was 'to take vows". When a person graduates in medicine, he/she takes a vow to serve the people.
- 'Vocation ': One expects to earn a living from service.
- 'Skilled': One has to develop skills in the area of service.
- 'Knowledge': The person is proficient in the body of knowledge.

Criteria of the Medical Profession

- The members of the medical profession possess a body of knowledge and skills in the field of medicine, over which its members have exclusive control.
- The work based on this knowledge is regulated by independent organizations.
- The mandate of these organizations is formalized by a variety of documents, including registration and licensure.
- The organizations serve as the ultimate authorities in medical practice.
- The profession determines the qualifications necessary to be a member of the profession, within the constraints of the law.
- The profession is responsible to ensure that the members follow the ethical and technical criteria; it has the right to discipline the unprofessional conduct.
- Members exhibit high standards of behaviour.
- The profession has a code of ethics, based on agreed values; members must 'do what is right and not do wrong'.

Recent Trends

The medical profession was considered to be a 'noble' profession. The literature is full of noble deeds of the members of the profession. But it is now losing some of the respect and regards, it had enjoyed earlier.

Medicine in India today is regarded as:

- being overly protective of its own rights, status and income;
- guilty of ignoring the wider social problems;
- inherently conservative; and
- failing to regulate itself effectively
  - protecting unethical and incompetent colleagues;
  - failing to accept responsibility for inequities in the health care system.

It is necessary for the professional associations, those responsible for the education of health professionals and for all the members of the profession to understand their role in society as healer-professional. There is need to encourage the ethical and intellectual growth of doctors by setting high standards of serving the society and maintaining the integrity of the profession.

ETHICAL PROBLEMS AND MEDICAL PROFESSION

There are a host of ethical problems facing the medical profession in India today. These concern mainly 3 areas.

1. Professional conduct of the doctors, in the patient-doctor, doctor-doctor and doctor-public relationships;
2. Ethical problems at the beginning and end of life; and
3. Problems of social justice and equity in health.

There are some emerging problems with respect to diseases, such as HIV/AIDS and alternative systems of medicine.

Problems Relating to Professional Conduct

1. Malpractices, negligence, unethical advertisements.
2. Irrational use of drugs. Unethical promotion of drugs.
3. Autonomy of patient vs paternalism, beneficence, non-maleficence.
4. Informed consent.
5. Confidentiality, privacy.
6. Use of sophisticated and costly technology.
7. Research, clinical trials, human experimentation.
8. Organ transplantation.
9. Conduct towards colleagues and peers and towards the public.

Problems Connected with the Beginning and End of Life

1. Genetics, genetic engineering, genetic manipulation, eugenics.
2. Right to life.
3. Control of fertility, contraception, abortion.
4. Sex-preselection, female foeticide, infanticide.
5. Assisted reproductive technology, artificial insemination by husband or donor, in vitro fertilization and embryo transfer, GIFT, surrogate mother.
6. Care of the terminally ill.

7. Euthanasia. The living will. Suicide.
8. Quality of life.

Problems Involving Social Justice and Equity in Health

1. Right to health.
2. Health policy. Vulnerable groups.
3. Equity. Distributive justice in health care.
4. Commercialisation of medical care.

CLINICAL ETHICS

Many medico-moral problems arise in the care of individual patients. Clinical ethics deals with them. These problems concern:
1. giving maximum benefits to the patient with the least risk (correct diagnosis and management of the patient, keeping the interests of the patient foremost),
2. needs of the patient and preferences of the patient (relatives/guardians) regarding their care,
3. costs to the patient, family and society, and
4. availability of resources.

Clinical ethics involves the meeting of two persons, which call for trust, integrity, competence, compassion and co-operation. Good clinical ethical decisions take into consideration:
1. well-defined indications for medical intervention,
2. patient (guardian/parent) preferences,
3. improvement in quality of life,
4. reduction of the burden on patient, family and society,
5. moral values, and
6. social and cultural factors.

In the patient-doctor relationships, there are many responsibilities placed on the doctor.
1. The patient requests for help, placing confidence and trust in the doctor. The doctor has to respond using medical knowledge, skills and attitude to the best of his ability to meet the needs of the patient. These call for:
   i. diagnosing as accurately as possible the patient's condition,
   ii. evaluation of the situation, including seriousness of the condition, need for interference (immediate or later), possible benefits and risks of alternative courses of action, and the physical, psychological and social impacts of the alternatives,

iii. making a clinical judgement as to the best course of action under the circumstances, and
iv. informing the patient (parent/guardian) as skillfully and accurately as possible about the patient's condition, the alternatives available, their benefits and risks and the best possible approach.

2. After considering all aspects, including patient preferences, the doctor carries out the procedures indicated.

A 28-year-old male came to the hospital with severe headache and stiffness of neck of recent onset. There were no localizing neurological signs. A provisional diagnosis of meningitis was made. A lumbar puncture was done. Bacteriological analysis of the cerebrospinal fluid showed that the patient had pneumococcal meningitis. The doctor informed the patient and suggested immediate treatment with an antibiotic. The patient refused. What shall the doctor do?

GOALS OF MEDICAL INTERVENTION

The classical aim of medical care has been "to cure sometimes, to relieve often, to comfort always". It brings out our limitations. In each patient, make a realistic assessment of the goals of management. These can be:

- restoration of complete health,
- relief of symptoms,
- maintenance of the compromised function, without further deterioration,
- saving life or prolonging life, and
- patient education and health education.

In all situations, avoid harm (nonmaleficence). The benefits must be always much more than the risks (favourable benefit/risk ratio).

In deciding on the goals, consider which goals are desirable and which are possible. The goals depend on:

1. nature of diseases,
2. options available,
3. preferences of the patient, and
4. social, cultural and economic factors.

In the patient with pneumococcal meningitis, the disease was acute and serious, which began abruptly. The diagnostic aid was simple. The lumbar puncture was done promptly and the cerebrospinal fluid analyzed. If the doctor had advised additionally a CT scan, it would have been inappropriate. It would also have been wrong if the hospital procedures delayed the performance of the lumbar puncture, analysis of the fluid and arriving at a diagnosis. The goal of complete restoration of health is desirable and possible.

The options available are good with a number of potent, yet not too costly, antibiotics which, applied in correct dose, can effect a cure. In this instance, social, cultural and economic factors do not present any ethical problems.

The patient preferred not to be treated by antibiotics. This has raised a problem. Sometimes it so happens that the patient refuses treatment but the patient's close relatives demand immediate treatment. Can the patient be given the treatment against his will?

A Chronic Disease with Acute Complication

Raman, aged 59 years, retired from Government service a year ago. He is an uncontrolled diabetic. He developed gangrene of the right foot and was admitted to the hospital. The doctor advised amputation below the knee as a life-saving measure. Raman refused. The doctor knows and explains to the patient that the best prognosis is by amputation. Otherwise it can be fatal. But the patient does not want to live with a compromised 'quality of life'. The patient goes into coma. The patient had made known his preference but his life is being threatened.

Should the doctor amputate the limb, even against the wishes of the patient and thus save his life? Will 'not doing' the operation amount to negligence or abetting suicide, should the patient die?

A Chronic Fatal Disease

Vimala, aged 33, has a critical disease, which is progressive, with remissions and exacerbations. The disease or its complication is fatal.

The goal of treatment is to retard disease and complications and alleviate the symptoms, e.g. pain.

The goal will also be to improve or preserve the limited function and help the patient retain dignity and sense of control of her life.

Ethical Problems

1. The progressive and critical deterioration of function seems to be leading to inevitable death. Should there be a goal of prolonging life?

   We cannot always say what the outcome of treatment will be. When there is any doubt, the advice would be to continue to treat.
2. During exacerbation, the condition could become very serious. The patient might have respiratory distress and may need resuscitation. There can be irreversible coma or brain death. Should the life support be continued? Can it be withdrawn? Many interventions are useful in the short run. If there is no improvement, there is no obligation to continue useless or futile interventions. But ordinary symptomatic relief must be provided, making the remaining part of the life as comfortable as possible.

A Chronic, Debilitating Disease

A 48-year-old female has rheumatoid arthritis. The condition is chronic with acute episodes. She is being treated in the clinic of the doctor but there is no definite cure. The goals of treatment are to (1) reduce pain, (2) prevent complications, (3) assist the patient live as comfortably as possible, and (4) provide patient and health education.

PATIENT-DOCTOR RELATIONSHIP

The patient-doctor relationship is in the nature of a special type of contract. Essential to the contract is the consent of both parties. The patient seeking medical care initiates the contract. When the doctor consents to provide care, the contract comes into being. The contract is sustained by the patient continuing to be under the care of the doctor. When the patient withdraws the consent, the contract is terminated.

The contract between the patient and the doctor is of a fiduciary relationship. The doctor is held responsible to a higher standard of performance than in an ordinary contract. The doctor, by virtue of his better knowledge and skills in the area of medical care, has an obligation to protect the best interests of the patient. The patient reposes trust and faith in the doctor. There is need for loyalty to the patient's interests. *Susruta Samhita* says:

> "The patient may doubt his relatives, his sons and even his parents but he has full faith in the physician. He gives himself up in the doctor's hand and has no misgivings about him. Therefore, it is the physician's duty to look after him as his own son".

Abandonment

"A physician is free to choose whom he will serve" states the Medical Council of India code of Ethics. Can the physician refuse to provide medical care? Theoretically, yes. But there can be situations when there is an obligation to serve, even though the physician is inclined not to. These arise in emergencies. Once the physician chooses to serve, he is not free to sever the professional relationship unilaterally without reasonable notice, at a time when there is still need for continued medical attention. A physician should not withdraw from the management of the patient without giving notice to the patient, his relatives or his responsible friends sufficiently in advance of his intention to withdraw to allow them to secure another medical attendant.

Conscientious Objection

A doctor may have conscientious objection to certain procedures, e.g. objection by a Catholic doctor to abortion. The hospital cannot force the doctor to perform an act against which the doctor has conscientious objections. So also, the hospital should make known their policies regarding practices (e.g. tubectomies, abortion), performed by others in the country generally but not allowed in the particular institution.

Bioethics

The recent advances in biology and medicine have produced and are producing innumerable ethical problems. Bioethics deals with such problems and distinguishes traditional medical ethics from these newer issues, arising out of advances in science and technology.

1. Applies ethical principles to the new and unsettling questions presented by scientific and technological advance which probe deep into the secrets of biology;
2. Determines whether there are unacceptable risks in technological development and scientific expertise;
3. Looks into the social aspects of health and health care as the equitable distribution of scientific achievement; and
4. Considers the principles of allocating scarce health resources, whether high-tech (organ transplants or in vitro fertilization), medium-tech (renal dialysis) or low-tech (primary health care).

Health Policy Ethics

These are concerned with ethical issues relevant to the health of the community. They deal with organizing, financing and delivery of healthcare services. Society has to ensure more equitable distribution of the benefits of medical knowledge and advances for the collective benefit of the present and future generations. This may call for social and economic control of the unrestrained use of resources and sophisticated technology in treating individual patients. Maximizing medical care for an individual may have to be given up in order to optimise health care for all.

Ideal Doctor

"The ideal doctor, one who respects his art, is never far from his patient. But those who practise for profit, since there is greater profit in a numerous clientele, gladly follow a school of teaching that does not demand such constant care"

—Cornelius Celsus, Rome, "On Medicine", nearly 2000 years ago.

CHAPTER 2

Teaching/Learning of Medical Ethics

Medical education today is characterized by vast knowledge base from cutting edge biomedical science to the professional artistry and high level of technical proficiency that students must acquire for practice. A physician needs to be prepared to work in relation with their patients and others in varied settings like clinics, hospitals and communities.

In India, selection of a student to a medical college is purely based on knowledge not taking into consideration the non-cognitive abilities of a student. So an Indian Medical Graduate (IMG) lags behind in communication skills and ethical literacy. Unfortunately very little learning in ethics takes place in the teaching institutions and doctors are not trained to analyze and solve ethical problems. Teaching of ethics calls attention to the implications of our actions, professional and personal.

Keeping the above factors in mind, fundamental changes in the Medical Education is the need of the hour. Hence to make MBBS curriculum more effective, MCI has proposed new teaching-learning approaches including a structured longitudinal program that help students to acquire non-cognitive competencies in addition to the basic knowledge of subjects.

The aim is to create an IMG who should have the knowledge of medico-legal, societal, ethical and humanitarian principles that greatly influence the health-care system. The development of ethical values and overall professional growth as integral part of curriculum shall be emphasized through a structured longitudinal program on professional development and ethics. MCI has allotted 40 hours for professional development including ethics in the foundation course of one month duration from the current session which is a welcome step.

Learning medical ethics starts with the anatomy laboratory (*Dissection Hall*). When a student enters the medical college, his first encounter is with the cadaver who act as "Silent Teachers". Respect for cadaver as a teacher translates later into respect for human beings as teachers and lifelong respect for learning. Throughout the world, the emphasis on humanizing the cadaver with respect as first patient or first teacher has gained momentum.

To inculcate the attitude of respect and gratitude from the very beginning, cadaveric oath should be taken by the undergraduate students which helps them to develop empathy with the cadaver and in the long run with the patients while serving the humanity by way of medical practice. Cadavers are gift by families to the medical colleges and anatomists are regarded as custodians of cadaveric material. Cadaver should be properly embalmed and stored. They should be properly covered with a cloth dipped in embalming fluid after every dissection. Anonymity of cadavers should be maintained. Tissues/visceras should be well preserved or stored in designated trays/containers. There should be safe disposal of biological tissue. An informed consent is must from families of donors for all images arising from cadavers for research purpose. This approach will help students to learn ethical values laying foundation for their clinical training.

The management of the patient often raises ethical problems, which need immediate attention. There will be many options. Ethically acceptable options must be selected and applied. A simple procedure like giving an antibiotic can become anethical issue (apart from technical issues depending on the infecting organism, sensitivity, age, adverse reactions, etc.) when the cost is so high that the patient/hospital/state cannot afford it and a cheaper alternative is available. In teaching clinical ethics, the goal is to develop the ability to:

- identify the underlying ethical issues and problems,
- consider the alternatives under the given circumstances, and
- make decisions, based on acceptable moral concepts as also traditions and practices.

In clinical ethics, a role model is very important, as also character building and skill acquisition. The clinician shows how the ethical principles are applied on a day-to-day and patient-to-patient basis. The clinician:

- demonstrates, by example, how to identify and resolve the particular problem,

- increases the awareness and knowledge of the student of the value dimensions of interactions with the patients, colleagues, relatives and public,
- fosters the development of skills of analysis, decisionmaking and judgement, and
- makes known to the student the need to respect the rights of the patient as also the duties and responsibilities of the doctor.

Just as in clinical medicine, the clinician may want to consult others knowledge able in ethics. They may be other clinicians or non-clinicians and even non-medical persons, such as sociologists, psychologists or anthropologists. They can bring in viewpoints which are different from that of the clinician. Together, it may be possible to tackle better the ethical problem of a particular patient or a group of patients. The ultimate decision will be that of the clinician.

Many of the larger hospitals have (or should have) ethics committees. Such committees will have knowledgeable members from different walks of life. It would be a good idea to involve the members of the committee in the framing of the curricula with respect to the teaching of ethics. Their involvement will enrich the program. Ethical problems are not easy to solve. Do not lose heart. The very fact that you find decision making difficult in certain situations shows your concern for the people. You are aware of the problem. Study the different facets of the problems. Study them in relation to the values. Do not give up saying that it is a difficult problem. It would not have been a problem if it was not difficult. There will be ethical dilemmas but if you are accustomed to analyze the problems, you will find that you can deal more competently with the tensions that develop and arrive at acceptable solutions.

Clinical ethics must be taught as part of the teaching of medical ethics. There will be case studies, problem analyzing and problem solving sessions, as also teaching and learning of the theoretical aspects. Classroom teachings will focus on professional relationships, patient-doctor relationships, issues at the beginning and end of life, reproductive technologies, allocation of resources and health policy. They will also deal with values, ethical concepts and principles.

Who will teach medical ethics? The clinician is a must. But his teaching can be supplemented by ethicists other than the clinicians. This will widen the horizon of the medical student.

The Medical Council of India recently initiated a reform that all medical students must be proficient in the knowledge and understanding of ethical and legal issues relevant to the practice of medicine. The council requires all the students to be able "to understand and analyze ethical problems so as to enable patients, their families, society and the doctor to have proper regard to such problems inreaching decisions".

Core Curriculum for Medical Ethics and Law (Adapted)

1. Informed consent and refusal of treatment
   - Respect for autonomy
   - Adequate information
   - Treatment without consent
   - Competence, battery, negligence
2. Truthfulness, trust and good communication
   - Building trust
   - Honesty; values in clinical practice
   - Communication skills
3. Confidentiality
   - Privacy
   - Compulsory/discretionary disclosure
   - Public-vs-private interest
4. Medical research
   - Regulation of medical research
   - Patients, volunteers, animals
5. Human reproduction
   - Embryo; fetus
   - Assisted conception
   - Abortion
   - Prenatal screening
6. Genetics
   - Treating the abnormal-*vs*-treating the normal
   - Genetic therapy and research
7. Children
   - Age to consent totreatment
   - Parental/child/clinician conflict
8. Mental disorders and disabilities
   - Detention and treatment with out consent
   - Conflicts of interests
   - Patient, family, community

9. Life, death, dying and killing
   - Life prolonging treatment
   - Life shortening palliatives
   - Transplantation
   - Death certification
10. Duties of doctors
   - Public expectation of medicine
   - Teamwork
   - GMC and professional regulation
   - Clinical mistakes
11. Resource allocation
   - "Rationing"
   - Equitable health care
   - Needs, utility, efficiency
12. Rights
   - Rights and links with moral and professional duties
   - Concepts of rights, including human rights.

St John's Medical College, Bengaluru

A rare exception to the neglect of the teaching of medical ethics in the country is St John's Medical College, Bengaluru. This institution started the teaching/learning of medical ethics from its inception. The institution has tried various methods of teaching ethics by the faculty of the institution and non-medical ethicists.

Rajiv Gandhi University of Health Sciences, Bengaluru

The recently established university has made the teaching/learning of medical ethics as part of the curriculum. This is unique among the universities in the country. The university conducted workshops on the teaching of medical ethics, so as to make the teaching effective.

TRAINING FOR TEACHERS IN MEDICAL ETHICS

It is essential to ensure that the teaching produces the desired results, as most of clinicians/other teachers are not proficient in the teaching of the subject.

The MCI has conducted workshops for faculty members on how to integrate ethical values into their curricula.

Objectives

- Increase the ethical sensitivity of students
- Increase the knowledge of relevant standards and codes of conduct
- Improve the ethical judgements
- Improve their ethical will power—their ability to live up to the highest ethical values.

Methods

- Study the literature on ethical values and then discuss them
- Guest lectures
- Films on ethical values and asking students to react
- Conduct regular courses on professional ethical conduct
- Make ethics pervade the entire curriculum.

It is essential to have similar workshops, wherever it is proposed to include the subject in the curriculum.

> "Life is short and the art long; the occasion fleeting; experience fallacious, and judgment difficult"
>
> —The Aphorisms, Hippocrates of Cos.

CHAPTER 3

Code of Conduct

Ethical codes of conduct are important for any profession. It is all the more so for the medical profession. The codes of conduct can succeed only if the profession, as a whole, feels responsible for its implementation. If the doctors as members of the profession fail to be responsible and do not take action against those who do not observe the code, the code becomes ineffective.

Ethical code is not legislation. But, it is equally forceful as it is approved by the profession. The final court in all actions is the conscience of the doctor (and of the patient). There appears a voice which summons the doctor to do what is good and avoid what is evil.

There are many Codes of Conduct. Among them are:

- *Atreya Anushasana*
- *Charaka Samhita*
- *Susruta Samhita*
- *Oath of Hippocrates*
- *International Code of Medical Ethics*
- *Medical Council of India, Code of Ethics*
  - Revised regulations, 2002.

HISTORICAL PERSPECTIVE

The first recorded code of conduct (according to *Ayurveda*) is the *Atreya Anushasana*.

Atreya Anushasana

If you desire success and fame as a physician:

1. you shall pray for the welfare of all creatures; day and night you shall endeavor to relieve their suffering with all your heart and soul;

2. you shall not injure nor desert your patient even for the sake of your own life or living;
3. you shall enter the patient's house after due permission, accompanied by a person known to him, bent of head and shall conduct yourself with utmost care and caution;
4. once inside the house, you shall devote your senses, mind and speech entirely to the patient, his ailments and things concerning him but shall not let them go astray;
5. you shall keep all information about the patient secret and shall not offend him by revealing it to others;
6. even if the patient's life was closing up, you shall not announce it either to him or to his relatives in a manner as would injure their feelings;
7. no offering of any kind, reward, present, eatables, etc. shall be accepted by you without the permission of the head of the family especially from the ladies without the knowledge and consent of their masters;
8. you shall conduct yourself dignified, respect the traditions and customs of the house, speak moderately, gently and rightly;
9. listen to and act suitably even to others, if it be for the benefit of the patient;
10. boast not your knowledge, though possessing it;
11. you shall be clean and modest in your attire and appearance;
12. you shall not commit adultery even in thought;
13. you shall not covet other's possessions and shall exercise restraint on your desires;
14. you shall not associate with sinners, drunkards, criminals and the mean nor shall act as their abettor;
15. reside not in places of ill-repute nor visit them;
16. harbour not jealousy towards elders, other physicians and respectables; regard them, consult them at times of doubt;
17. medical science is eternal and noble, follow it with diligence and faith, uphold its aims and by so doing attain happiness here and hereafter.

Charaka Samhita

Code of conduct for the would be physicians:

- Your action must be free from ego, vanity, worry, agitation of mind or envy; your actions must be carefully planned, with concern for the patient and in keeping with the instructor's advice.

- Your unceasing efforts must, at all costs (*sarvatmana*) be directed towards giving health to the suffering patients (*aturanam arogya*).
- You must never harbor feelings of ill-will towards your patients, whatever the provocation, even if it entails risk to your life.
- Never should you entertain thoughts (*manasapi*) of sexual misconduct or thoughts of appropriating property that does not belong to you.
- Take no liquor, commit no sin, nor keep company with the wicked.
- Your speech must be soft, pleasant, virtuous, truthful, useful and moderate.
- What you do must be appropriate to the place where you practice and the time and you must be mindful in whatever you do?
- Your efforts must be unremitting (*nityam yatnavata cha*).
- Do not reveal to others what goes on in the patients' household (*aturakula pravarthayah*).
- Even when you are learned and proficient, do not show off.

Susruta Samhita

Susruta Samhita, which is equally ancient also gives guidelines particularly with respect to surgeons and surgical procedures. Vagabhata, the elder says "Friendship with all, sympathy towards the sick, feeling of profound satisfaction upon recovery and overlooking even those who have ill-will towards him are sufficient to fulfill the ethical requirements of a doctor".

Another ancient code of conduct for doctors is contained in the *Hippocratic Oath*. It is in the form of an oath and therefore binding on the person.

Oath of Hippocrates

"I swear by Apollo Physician, by Aesclepeus, by Hygiea, by Panacea and by all the gods and goddesses, making them my witnesses that I will carry out, according to my ability and judgement, this oath and indenture.

To hold my teacher in this art equal to my own parents; to make him partner in my livelihood; where he is in need of money to share mine with him; to consider his family as my own brothers, and to teach them this art, if they want to learn it, without fee or indenture.

To impart precept, oral instruction, and all other instructions to my own sons, the sons of my teacher and to indentured pupils who have taken the physician's oath, but to nobody else.

I will use treatment to help the sick according to my ability and judgement, but never with a view to injury and wrong-doing. Neither will I administer a poison to anybody when asked to do so, nor will I suggest such a course. Similarly, I will not give to a woman a pessary to cause abortion. But I will keep pure and holy both my life and my art.

I will not use the knife, not even verily on sufferers from stone, but I will give place to such as are craftsmen therein.

Into whatsoever houses I enter, I will enter to help the sick and I will abstain from all intentional wrong-doing and harm, especially from abusing the bodies of man or woman, bond or free.

And whatsoever I shall see or hear in the course of my profession, as well as outside my profession in my intercourse with men, if it be what should not be published abroad, I will never divulge, holding such things to be holy secrets.

Now, if I carry out this oath and break it not, may I gain for ever reputation among all men for my life and for my art; but if I transgress it and forswear myself, may the opposite befall me.

The *Hippocratic Oath* is based on Greek tradition. It continues to influence even today. But changes were seen to be necessary and we have other declarations.

There does not appear to be any articulated ancient code of medical ethics according to the Chinese tradition. Confucianism and Buddhism regulated all activities including medical practice. Sun Simiao published a treatise *"On the Absolute Sincerity of Great Physicians"* (called the Chinese Hippocratic Oath) in his work titled *"The Important Prescriptions Worth a Thousand Pieces of Gold"*. According to this treatise, the physician should:

1. develop first the sense of compassion and piety,
2. commit himself to make effort to save every living creature,
3. treat every patient on equal grounds, and
4. not seek wealth by his expertise.

There was no code of conduct, as such, until 1937, when *"The Creed for Doctors"* was published by the Chinese Association of Doctors. After the communists came to power, the tenets of communism became the guiding principles.

A conference on "Philosophy of Medicine" held in Canton in 1979 focused on two issues in medical ethics: Concept of death and euthanasia and delivery of medical care without discrimination.

INTERNATIONAL CODE OF MEDICAL ETHICS (1983)

A Physician shall always maintain the highest standards of professional conduct.

A Physician shall not permit motives of profit to influence the free and independent exercise of professional judgement on behalf of patients.

A Physician shall, in all types of medical practice, be dedicated to providing competent medical service in full technical and moral independence with compassion and respect for human dignity.

A Physician shall deal honestly with patients and colleagues, and strive to expose those physicians deficient in character or competence or who engage in fraud or deception. The following practices are deemed to be unethical conduct:

a. Self advertising by physicians, unless permitted by the law of the country and the Code of Ethics of the National Medical Association.
b. Paying or receiving any fee or any other consideration solely to procure the referral of a patient or for prescribing or referring a patient to any source.

A Physician shall respect the rights of colleagues, and of other professionals, and shall safeguard patient confidence.

A Physician shall act only in the patient's interest when providing medical care which might have the effect of weakening the physical and mental condition of the patient.

A Physician shall use great caution in divulging discoveries or new techniques or treatment through non-professional channels.

A Physician shall certify only that which he has personally verified.

Duties of Physicians to the Sick

A Physician shall always bear in mind the obligation of preserving human life.

A Physician shall owe his patients complete loyalty and all the resources of his science. Whenever an examination or treatment is beyond the physician's capacity he should summon another physician who has the necessary ability.

A Physician shall preserve absolute confidentiality on all he knows about his patient even after the patient has died.

A Physician shall give emergency care as a humanitarian duty unless he is assured that others are willing and able to give such care.

Duties of Physicians to Each Other

A Physician shall behave towards his colleagues as he would have them behave towards him.

A Physician shall not entice patients from his colleagues.

A Physician shall observe the principles of the 'Declaration of Geneva' approved by the World Medical Association.

THE INDIAN MEDICAL COUNCIL ACT, 1956

Section 20A: Professional Conduct

1. The Council may prescribe professional conduct and etiquette and a code of ethics for medical practitioners.
2. Regulations made by the Council under sub-section (1) may specify which violations thereof shall constitute infamous conduct in any professional respect, that is to say, professional misconduct, and such provision shall have effect not withstanding anything contained in any law for the time being in force (Inserted by Act 24 of 1964).

As per the above section under the Indian Medical Council Act, 1956, the Medical Council of India published the Code of Medical Ethics and this was approved by the Central Government in 1970. This has been revised and issued as "the Indian Medical Council (Professional Conduct, Etiquette and Ethics) Regulations, 2002". It was published in the Gazette of India Part III, Section 4, dated 6th April, 2002 and the Regulations have come into force. (Please see Annexure I for the Regulations).

CHAPTER 4 Malpractice and Negligence

Malpractice is professional misconduct. There is failure in carrying out the professional duties with competence and integrity, in the "best interests" of the patient. There may be improper or insufficient knowledge and skills, or their defective application, or wrong attitude. The accepted norms of care must be exercised. Substandard management of the patient, whether due to incompetence, negligence or ulterior motives, is a breach of duty. Every doctor has a duty to prevent malpractice. The code of Ethics of the Medical Council of India says: "A physician should expose without fear or favour, incompetent or corrupt, dishonest or unethical conduct on the part of the members of the profession".

INCOMPETENCE

Quality assurance is a must in medical care. The most important factor in assuring quality is the competence of the doctor.

Competence of the doctor is determined first when he/she

i. undergoes the prescribed course of study,
ii. satisfies the examiners,
iii. does the internship to the satisfaction of the authorities, and
iv. gets registered by the Medical Council.

The doctor is licensed to practise, being considered to have the required competence to provide medical care. Will the doctor continue to be competent thereafter? Will the doctor continue to acquire the newer knowledge and skills brought on by the advances in medical sciences? If he/she does not cope with the advances, the quality of care suffers and does not measure up to the standards expected. Many doctors tend to deteriorate, over a period of time, in their knowledge, skills and attitude. Not only do they not make any attempt to update themselves but they slip down.

How can we determine whether the doctor continues to meet the appropriate standards of general or speciality practice?

At present, we do not have any system in India to ensure continued competence. Some countries have periodical re-registration. We can help the doctor to maintain competence. Continuing medical education can make available the needed knowledge, attitude and skills, with awareness of the advances in medicine. If the doctor makes use of it deligently, continuing medical education can help to build up adequate competence to discharge his/her duties. It is not difficult to assess knowledge. It is not that easy to assess skills. It is extremely difficult to measure other critical characteristics so important in patient care, integrity, respect for the patient, compassion, cost containment and others.

MEDICAL PRACTITIONERS' FITNESS TO PRACTISE

Many medical practitioners continue to practise medicine even when they are not in a fit condition to practise.

Impaired physician is one who is unable to practise medicine with reasonable skill and safety to patients because of physical and mental illness due to various causes including the ageing process, loss of motor skills, or excessive use or abuse of drugs including alcohol. Mentally impaired physicians may experience erosion of professional competence and can pose danger to their patients.

Doctors are subject to increasing emotional problems. Close encounter with death may disturb the doctor; so also fear of making a mistake or having made a mistake and the possibility of legal complaint or negligence suit and investigation. Ready availability of drugs and ability to afford alcohol can be contributing causes. Depression may arise from too much workload. Hospitalization rates due to psychiatric causes are more common in USA among male doctors than their counterparts belonging to same social class. The common causes are alcoholism, drug dependence and affective disorders.

Doctors may become incompetent due to many cuases:

> Shankar (name changed) is a general practitioner. He had been a good and competent practitioner, loved and respected by his patients, his colleagues and all in the neighborhood. He has now become old and forgetful. Some of his colleagues would like him to stop practice but do not wish to tell him so. Many of his diagnoses are wrong, prescriptions are often of no use and sometimes harmful.

What is to be done in case of incompetence? Individual doctors, professional associations and the state should come forward to help the impaired (incompetent) doctor, with empathy. In the case of Dr Shankar, one specialist took courage and over a cup of tea, apprised Dr Shankar of the situation. Dr Shankar said: "I did not know; no one told me". He promptly stopped his practice, following the ethical principle: First of all, do not harm.

Programs must be established to identify and help the impaired doctor. Counseling services must be available, it must be voluntary and confidentially maintained. Active participation of 'sick' doctor must be sought and obtained. Progress must be monitored, especially in instances of alcohol and drug abuse. It is the duty of the members of the medical profession to take steps to ensure that standards of care are kept up. The code of conduct requires it.

NEGLIGENCE

> "Negligence is the omission to do something which a reasonable man, guided upon those considerations which ordinarily regulate the conduct of human affairs, would do, or doing something which a prudent and reasonable man would not do"
>
> —Salmond, Law of Torts.

The doctor-patient relationship is in the form of an implied contract. It comes into existence when:

- a patient seeks the professional services of the doctor, and
- the doctor agrees to undertake the care of the patient.

This relationship places a responsibility on the doctor to:
- act in accordance with the established standards of the medical profession,
- take all reasonable care of the patient, and
- avoid all unreasonable risks.

The standard of care required is that of an ordinary skilled person, professing to have and exercising the knowledge and skill at that level (general or specialist) of service. A reasonable degree of care and competence must be exercised, as judged in the light of the circumstances of the case. The highest degree of care is not required; the lowest degree of care is not enough. If the doctor fails to measure up to the expected standard of care, the doctor is negligent. If as a result of negligence, harm is done, the doctor is liable to pay damages.

The principle of negligence applies whether the doctor:
- accepts fees or not;
- is in private practice or employed; or
- is a general practitioner or a specialist.

If employed, the employer may have vicarious responsibility. The doctor has a duty of care in:
- deciding whether to accept the patient for treatment (though it is maintained that the doctor is free to accept or reject a patient, there are circumstances where this freedom is questioned);
- deciding on the various aspects of diagnosis and management; and
- administering the treatment.

A woman with complicated pregnancy was advised by the primary health center to go to the District Hospital. On her way in an autorickshaw, she had labor pains and went to a private clinic on the way. The doctor refused to take the patient saying that he is not experienced in obstetrics and that he is not equipped to deal with labor cases. The woman delivered on the roadside. There was a public outcry and the doctor was arrested.

If there is a breach of duty of care, then the doctor is negligent. The standard can vary:
- from time to time (advances in medical care);
- with the situation (availability of tests and infrastructure); and
- if the doctor is a general practitioner or a specialist.

Error in diagnosis or treatment may occur. The doctor is not liable for negligence if the doctor has acted in accordance with the accepted medical practice in the given circumstances. The doctor-patient contract is a commitment of deed and not of the final result.

Many instances of negligence occur.

Nagamma, 38 years, had an operation for an ovarian cyst. After going home, she developed pain. Pus began coming out through an opening in the scar. She was operated again. An artery forceps and a piece of guaze were found within the abdomen.

Blood of wrong group was transfused to a patient without cross-matching. She developed renal failure and died.

A patient was admitted for elective surgery. The surgeon asked for a blood transfusion as the hemoglobin level was low. The blood was transfused before the results of the Australia antigen test came. The donor blood tested positive.

A doctor is negligent, if:

- the performance of the doctor falls below the standard of a reasonably competent practitioner at that level,
- there is negligence in diagnosis, administration of drugs or procedures including operations,
- there is failure to take all reasonable precautions, or
- there is any other kind of negligence in providing care.

Most of the cases of negligence do not come to the notice of the public or the law. But increasing numbers of doctors are now being taken to the court and damages are being awarded. To establish negligence, there must be a reasonable connection between the act or failure to act by the doctor, and harm caused to the patient. For the award of damages, actual injury or damage must be caused and proved to be so caused.

There are many pronouncements by the courts (and award of damages) in this country and much more so abroad.

Peter Pain, J (1983): "A doctor owed a duty to his patient to observe the precautions which were normal in the course of the treatment that he gave".

McNair, J (1959): "In the case of a medical man, negligence means failure to act in accordance with the standards of reasonably competent medical man at that time. That is a perfectly accurate statement as long as it is remembered that there may be one or more perfectly proper standards; and if a medical man conforms with one of those proper standards, then he is not negligent".

Lord Denning (1954) stated in *Hatcher-vs-Black*: "When a person who is ill, goes in for treatment, there is always some risk, no matter what care is used. Every surgical operation involves risks. It would be wrong, and indeed bad law, to say that simply because a misadventure or mishap occurred, the hospital and doctors are thereby liable".

Many doctors take insurance against claims of negligence and damages. But that is not enough. The medical profession must be alert. Doctors must take steps to prevent negligence. The Royal College of Surgeons and the Faculty of Anaesthetists, UK, conducted a confidential enquiry into operative deaths. The finding of the (Dr Brendan Devlin) committee was that about a thousand patients die in a year through errors in the operation theater in UK. The failure rates are much higher when the operation is done by "Occasional operators".

If death occurs on the operative table, who is responsible? Surgeon, Anaesthetist, or the hospital/nursing home?

When death occurs on the table, it is the duty of the surgeon and/or the hospital authorities to inform the police (or coroner, where applicable). They will make the necessary investigations and decide if the patient died a natural death or due to negligence. Action will be taken accordingly. The operation theaters must have adequate facilities.

There is a time limit for lodging complaints which may be civil or criminal. It is three years for civil complaints. For criminal law, it is up to two years. In the case of a minor, complaints can be filed 2/3 years after the minor reaches eighteen years of age. Criminal action can be taken in case of wrong diagnosis, mismatched blood transfusion or if the monitor is not working. Fraud, like charging costs for services not rendered, can be sued under civil law.

Where a claim is brought for the tort, damage is a necessary element of the cause of action. If the plaintiff fails to prove that any loss or injury was caused by the negligence, then he/she will not be entitled to damages.

Sueing under criminal law will be according to the Indian Penal Code sections 304A, 336, 337 and 338. Section 304A states: "Whosoever causes death of any person by any rash and negligent act not amounting to culpable homicide, shall be punished".

Section 336 states: "Whoever does any act so rashly or negligently as to endanger human life or the personal safety of others shall be punished". Similarly, sections 337 and 338 provide for punishment when hurt is caused by rash or negligent acts.

The Consumer Protection Act, 1986, provides for obtaining relief for any person "who hires any services for a consideration which has been paid or promised, partly paid and promised or under any system of deferred payments and includes any beneficiary of such services_____".

PROFESSIONAL CERTIFICATES

An area where there is considerable amount of unethical conduct is the issue of professional certificates. For a small fee or because of pressures, some doctors issue false certificates. All doctors must abide by the guidelines given by the Medical Council of India.

"Registered practitioners are in certain cases bound by law to give or may from time to time be called upon or requested to give certificates, notification, reports and other documents of similar character signed by them in their professional capacity for subsequent use in the courts of justice or for administrative purpose, etc.

"Any registered practitioner who shall be known to have signed or given under his name and authority any such certificate, notification, report or document of a similar character which is untrue, misleading or improper is liable to have his name erased from the Register"—Indian Medical Council Regulations, 2002.

> Mr Ram, aged about 50 years, approached Dr Narayan for a disability certificate to get some disability pension from the Government. Dr Narayan assessed the disability at 25% and issued a certificate. The patient went away but returned 2 days later with a powerful local leader, who demanded that the certificate be changed to 40% disability, with which alone Mr Ram can get the pension. The doctor was in a dilemma. He was sympathetic and wanted to help. At the same time, his assessment according to all the norms was that the disability was only 25%.
>
> What should Dr Narayan do?

REBATES AND COMMISSION

There are complaints especially in the cities and larger towns that dubious arrangements are made by doctors by which patients have to pay unnecessarily, with profits going to the doctors involved. There seems to be a growing tendency for making more and more referrals for diagnostic tests and consultations. Where they are truly indicated such referrals are beneficial to the patient. Occasionally, they are done because of 'kick-backs'. Such referrals for personal gains, direct or indirect, are unethical.

"A physician shall not give, solicit or receive nor shall he offer to give, solicit, or receive any gift, gratuity, commission or bonus in consideration of or in return for the referring, recommending or procuring of any patient for medical, surgical or other treatment. A physician shall not directly or indirectly participate in or be a party to the acts of divisions, transference, assignment, subordination, rebating, splitting or refunding of any fee for medical, surgical or other treatment.

"These provisions shall apply with equal force to the referring, recommending or procuring by a physician or any person, specimen or material for diagnostic or other study or work".

—Indian Medical Council Regulations, 2002.

Such referrals, splitting and sharing seem to be prevalent in all countries. Bob Hope, in his characteristic jocular way, says: "I do not know whether my doctor is a physican or a booking agent. All that he does is to book appointments with other physicians".

ADVERTISING AND PROMOTION

An unfortunate trend is the increasing violation by some of the doctors of the code of ethical conduct which prohibited or limited advertising. With the modern tendency for aggressive advertising, some doctors seem to consider that they can also indulge in unethical advertising.

The code of Ethics of the Medical Council of India says:

"Solicitation of patients directly or indirectly by a physician, by groups of physicians or by institutions or organisations is unethical".

"A Physician shall not make use of or aid or permit others to make use of him or his name as subject of any form or manner of advertising or publicity through any mode either alone or in conjunction with others which is of such a character as to invite attention to him.........

"Nor shall he boast of cases, operations, cures or remedies or permit the publication of report thereof through any mode".

A medical practitioner is permitted a formal announcement in the press on:

1. starting practice,
2. change of type of practice,
3. change of address,
4. temporary absence from duty,
5. resumption of practice, and
6. succeeding to another practice.

Accepting Gifts

Gift-giving and receiving are rampant. The manufacturers/producers want to persuade the doctor to prescribe certain products. Very often this leads to the prescription of unnecessarily costly drugs, without proper indication or assessment. Inducements are of various kinds. They may be in the nature of pens, calenders, diaries, desk stands or beautiful paper weights with the name of the firm/product printed or embossed. It may be in the nature of invitations to lunches or dinners,preceded by "scientific discussions". Companies may host conferences, "all in the interests of better patient care". Invitations are given to the specialists/consultants/administrators to spend weekends in Singapore or other lovely distant places, all expenses paid, "discussing - scientifically, of course—the merits of the particular product".

Some doctors avoid the question whether these are ethical ways of promotion of drugs, equipment or other products. They say that "I may accept the gifts but I take my own decisions". Are the firms so foolish?

UNNECESSARY PROCEDURES

There is a general feeling that some doctors indulge in unnecessary procedures, whether they be operative procedures or prescribing drugs. Often such procedures are of doubtful value and may even be harmful. One such procedure used to be appendicectomy. Fortunately, it is on the decrease. Prescribing multivitamin preparations and tonics, without any indication whatsoever, still continues.

Kalyani, 22 years, delivered normally a 3 kg baby. Both mother and child were healthy. Next day, the mother was given an intravenous infusion of dextrose to which was added a multivitamin preparation. There was an anaphylactic reaction and the mother died.

The insert for the multivitamin preparation contained in small letters, a warning that hypersensitivity reaction may occur in 1 in 10,000 persons.

The obstetrician was asked why the dextrose and multivitamin preparation were given. The answer was "we always give". There was no indication whatsoever.

Because of this unnecessary procedure, the child became a one-parent child, losing the mother's care. The young father became a widower.

Sometimes the procedures are unnecessarily costly. This is especially so with "confirmatory" tests. Doctors must determine whether the particular procedure (diagnostic or treatment) is indicated and whether it is the best alternative (considering the benefits, risks and cost) among those available.

Questionable increases have been occurring in the number of cesarian sections and hysterectomies.

Participation in Torture

An extreme instance of malpractice is participation in torture. The doctor may not be quite aware of such participation initially. That was what happened in Nazi Germany. Doctors began participating in "human experimentation" and "eugenics" which later on became torture and extermination of certain races.

The doctor's participation in torture may be in various ways:

1. Assessing the victim's health before torture, to ascertain whether the victim is 'fit' to be tortured;
2. Determining how much longer it is possible to continue the torture without killing the victim;
3. Reviving the victim who has collapsed or has been rendered unconscious by the torture; and
4. Actively participating in the process.

Such tortures go on every day, whether it is by the police or by the terrorists. Most often the victim is tortured to extract information or a "confession". Participation in torture or even in interrogation of the prisoner or victim is unethical.

THE DECLARATION OF TOKYO (WMA, 1975)

The Declaration of Tokyo has since its adoption in 1975, been the most comprehensive statement produced by the medical profession on the question of the torture and cruel, inhuman or degrading treatment of detainees. It was adopted by the 29th World Medical Assembly, Tokyo, Japan.

Declaration of Tokyo

It is the privilige of the medical doctor to practice medicine in the service of humanity, to preserve and restore bodily and mental health without distinction as to persons, to comfort and to ease the suffering of his or her patients. The utmost respect for human life is to be maintained even under threat, and no use made of any medical knowledge contrary to the laws of humanity.

For the purpose of this Declaration, torture is defined as the deliberate, systematic or wanton infliction of physical or mental suffering by one or more persons acting alone or on the orders of any authority, to force another person to yield information, to make a confession, or for any other reason.

1. The doctor shall not countenance, condone or participate in the practice of torture or other forms of cruel, inhuman or degrading procedures, whatever the offence of which the victim of such procedures is suspected, accused or guilty, and whatever the victim's beliefs or motives, and in all situations, including armed conflict and civil strife.
2. The doctor shall not provide any premises, instruments, substances or knowledge to facilitate the practice of torture or other forms of cruel, inhuman or degrading treatment or to diminish the ability of the victim to resist such treatment.
3. The doctor shall not be present during any procedure during which torture or other forms of cruel, inhuman or degrading treatment is used or threatened.
4. A doctor must have complete clinical independence in deciding upon the care of a person for whom he or she is medically responsible. The doctor's fundamental role is to alleviate the distress of his/her fellow men, and no motive whether personal, collective or political shall prevail against this higher purpose.
5. Where a prisoner refuses nourishment and is considered by the doctor as capable of forming an unimpaired and rational

judgment concerning the consequences of such a voluntary refusal of nourishment, he or she shall not be fed artificially. The decision as to the capacity of the prisoner to form such a judgment should be confirmed by at least one other independent doctor. The consequences of the refusal of nourishment shall be explained by the doctor to the prisoner.

6. The World Medical Association will support, and should encourage the international community, the national medical associations and fellow doctors, to support the doctor and his or her family in the face of threats or reprisals resulting from a refusal to condone the use of torture or other forms of cruel, inhuman or degrading treatment.

PRINCIPLES OF MEDICAL ETHICS (UNITED NATIONS, 1982)

The principles are elaborated within the text of Resolution 37/194 adopted by the United Nations General Assembly, 18th December 1982.

The Geneal Assembly...

DESIROUS of setting further standards in this field which ought to be implemented by health personnel, particularly physicians, and by government officials.

1. ADOPTS the Principles of Medical Ethics relevant to the role of health personnel, particularly physicians, in the protection of prisoners and detainees against torture and other cruel, inhuman or degrading treatment or punishment set forth in the annex to the present resolution;
2. CALLS UPON all governments to give the Principles of Medical Ethics, together with the present resolution, the widest possible distribution, in particular among medical and paramedical associations and institutions of detention or imprisonment in an official language of the State;
3. INVITES all relevant inter-governmental organizations, in particular the World Health Organization, and non-governmental organizations concerned to bring the Principles of Medical Ethics to the attention of the widest possible group of individuals, especially those active in the Medical and paramedical field.

Principles of medical ethics relevant to the role of health personnel, particularly physicians, in the protection of prisoners and detainees against torture and other cruel, inhuman or degrading treatment or punishment

PRINCIPLE 1

Health personnel, particularly physicians, charged with the medical care of prisoners and detainees have a duty to provide them with protection of their physical and mental health and treatment of disease of the same quality and standard as is afforded to those who are not imprisoned or detained.

PRINCIPLE 2

It is a gross contravention of medical ethics, as well as an offence under applicable international instruments, for health personnel, particularly physicians, to engage, actively or passively, in acts which constitute participation in, complicity in, incitement to or attempts to commit torture or other cruel, inhuman or degrading treatment or punishment.

PRINCIPLE 3

It is a contravention of medical ethics for health personnel, particularly physicians, to be involved in any professional relationship with prisoners or detainees the purpose of which is not solely to evaluate, protect or improve their physical and mental health.

PRINCIPLE 4

It is a contravention of medical ethics for health personnel, particularly physicians:

a. to apply their knowledge and skills in order to assist in the interrogation of prisoners and detainees in a manner that may adversely affect the physical or mental health or condition of such prisoners or detainees and which is not in accordance with the relevant international instruments;
b. to certify, or to participate in the certification of, the fitness of prisoners or detainees for any form of treatment or punishment that may adversely affect their physical or mental health and which is not in accordance with the relevant international

instruments, or to participate in any way in the infliction of any such treatment or punishment which is not in accordance with the relevant international instruments.

PRINCIPLE 5

It is a contravention of medical ethics for health personnel, particularly physicians, to participate in any procedure for restraining a prisoner or detainee unless such a procedure is determined in accordance with purely medical criteria as being necessary for the protection of the physical or mental health or the safety of the prisoner or detainee himself, or his fellow prisoners or detainees, or of his guardians, and presents no hazard to his physical or mental health.

PRINCIPLE 6

There may be no derogation from the foregoing principles on any grounds whatsoever, including public emergency.

CHAPTER 5

Confidentiality (Professional Secrecy)

Confidentiality is part of the larger issue of a patient's privacy. Every patient is entitled to privacy. Confidentiality is informational privacy. The individual has the right to determine how, when and to what extent data about self will be released to another person. Doctor is given confidential information which is not to be passed on to a third party. There is implicit understanding and undertaking as to what the doctor will do with the information to treat fully the patient with the illness. If confidences are broken, patients may not give full information; it can be detrimental to proper diagnosis and treatment. Matters confided to the doctor in the course of the professional relationship between the doctor and the patient must not be divulged to others. The oaths and declarations taken or made by the doctor insist on informational secrecy.

> "All that may come to my knowledge in the exercise of my profession or outside of my profession or in daily commerce with me which ought not to be spread abroad, I will keep secret and will never reveal"
>
> -Hippocratic oath

> "I will respect the secrets which are confided in me even after the patient has died"
>
> -Geneva declaration

Individuals value their privacy. It must be respected.

Breaches in confidentiality might occur under a variety of situations:

- gossiping between doctors or the doctor and others;

- leaving notes on the desk, where it is accessible to others not directly involved in patient care;
- press and employer's representatives may pose as close relatives and ask for information
- talks over telephone.

There is need for safeguards:

- when approached by lawyers, employers, and insurance companies;
- computer-held records;
- when collecting health statistics.

Information may be given to a third party in certain situations. Even in such instances, as far as possible, obtain the consent of the patient to the disclosure.

- Notifiable infectious diseases (to the designated health authority).
- Infectious diseases, where the person with the disease is a risk to the community, e.g. typhoid carrier, who is a food handler.
- Risk to public safety, e.g. a driver who is color blind.
- Injury resulting from a suspected criminal act (Police to be informed).
- Disclosure necessitated in the court.
- When required by law (state regulations) and as an expert witness in the court.

Problems arise when there is the possibility of serious harm to an innocent third party, e.g. in the case of sexually transmitted diseases, which may be transmitted to the spouse. This has become a major problem with human immunodeficiency virus infection. There are also instances when the good of the patient requires it, e.g. when the patient threatens to commit suicide. In such instances, the doctor must make judicious decision in the best interest of the patient and the third party.

Confidentiality must be maintained in the publication of case reports. All reputed journals take care of it.

Many categories of people request for information: Insurance companies, prospective employers and others. Do not reveal personal information about the individual, unless a written release is obtained from the person.

An organization 'Q' has an arrangement with hospital 'H' for the referral of their employees for treatment. Patient 'P' was referred and had the treatment. The bill was sent to the organization, who paid the bill. They wanted full information on the patient. The hospital refused to divulge the matter, stating that the matter is confidential between the patient and the doctor/hospital. They said that only if the patient gives the clearance will the information be given. The organization was unhappy and terminated the arrangement with the hospital.

There is confidentiality of all medical records. There is a demand that access be given to medical records. Modern methods of storage of information in computers can lead to violation of confidentiality. Special precautions must be taken to limit access to information only to those involved in patient care and bound by confidentiality.

Confidentiality must be maintained when we discuss matters with others regarding the patient. These may be other members of the health team or employees of the hospital. It is important to ensure that they also do not tell others what has been written or discussed. When sharing the case files with others, care must be exercised to ensure confidentiality. It is also necessary to maintain confidentiality while presenting cases before conferences and other audiences.

In addition to informational privacy, there is need for physical privacy (e.g. while undressing for physical examination or for carrying out various procedures), psychological privacy and social privacy.

CHAPTER 6

Autonomy and Informed Consent

AUTONOMY

Doctors in India have been accustomed to take decisions on behalf of the patient, as to what should be done when a patient is in need of medical help. Medical practice has been traditionally paternalistic. We tend to justify paternalism by the concern of the doctor for the welfare and happiness of the patient. When the patient is ill, we think that the patient will not be in a position to make correct decisions. The patient does not know what the specialist knows. Doctors, patients and public often assume that "the doctor knows best", because of his or her qualifications, training and experience. There has been trust in the "goodness" of the doctor.

In recent times, a change has been coming, influenced by western thought. There is increasing conflict between the older *ethics of trust* and the *ethics of rights*. The ethics of trust held sway because of the conduct of the doctor to the patients and the patient's implicit faith in the doctor. In India, ethics of trust still holds good to a very large extent but there is increasing demand for ethics of rights. In the western world, ethics of rights is dominant.

> "Every human being of adult years and of sound mind has a right to determine what shall be done to his/her body".

Each person is master of his/her own body and has every right to object to the performance of any procedure he/she does not approve. There is need for consent. The consent must be based on adequate information. Such consent has to be documented.

Autonomy denotes the freedom of the patient (person) to determine what shall be done to him/her. There is the right to self-determination.

An informed preference of the patient (person) who is competent must be respected.

The right of choice is with the patient. A person can exercise his/her choice only if he/she has adequate knowledge of the options available and the benefits and risks involved in each of the alternatives. The doctor has to supply all the information. The doctor cannot substitute his/her own judgement about the best interests of the patient.

Supreme Court of Canada (114 DLR 3d 1)

Patient R had been suffering from headache and had high blood pressure. Dr H recommended the removal of a plaque in the left carotid artery. The patient wanted to know the details. The doctor assured the patient that if the operation is done, the patient will be alright and can go back to work in ten days' time. The operation was done. Patient had a massive stroke leading to paralysis on one side. The court awarded damages on the following basis:

- there was not enough disclosure of the risks involved in the operation;
- enough information was not given of the alternatives;
- there was negligence.

The court, while awarding damages, said: "The courts cannot stand idly by, if the medical profession by an excess paternalism, denies its patients a real choice. In a word, the law will not permit the medical profession to play God".

Competence

Autonomy raises the question of competence of the patient (person) to make appropriate decisions. The patient must be able to:

- understand the nature of the diseases and its consequences,
- analyse the problem,
- choose between the alternatives, and
- make a decision.

Competence may be lacking in a patient who is:

- too young (developmental incapacity),
- disoriented or confused (too old or due to disease or injury; mentally retarded), or
- mentally ill (psychotic).

The patient must possess the sensory and mental powers to process the information, data and the conclusions. The deficits may be temporary or permanent.

If autonomy is based on competence of the patient, it becomes necessary to determine whether the patient is competent. How can we assess competence? Many tests can be done to evaluate the competence:

Assess the orientation of the patient to the place, time, person and situation.

- Test memory—recent and past
- Observe for logical sequencing
- Assess intellectual capacity
- Assess the behavior of the patient. Is the patient agitated, anxious or showing evidence of abnormal behavior?
- Review past history for psychotic disturbances including drug history.

Any one of the above tests by itself alone is inadequate. Make an overall assessment. It will give a more correct picture of the person.

Autonomy of one person can affect the health of others, as in the case of infectious diseases. There is risk of spread of infection. So also, if some persons refuse immunization, it can affect the 'herd' immunity.

Can a patient harm himself or herself by refusing treatment? Will it amount to suicide? Will the doctor be assisting suicide by going along with the patient's decision not to take the proposed treatment, which could be life-saving?

Can a person's autonomy extend to the freedom of smoking as he/she desires? Passive smoking by others in the vicinity can cause diseases.

The Patient Self Determination Act of USA, enacted following the 1990 US Supreme Court decision, acknowledges the patient's right to direct healthcare decisions. The patient can give advance directives as to what should be done in given circumstances. The patient can accept or refuse medical treatment. Even artificial provision of nutrition and/or hydration is considered medical treatment and the person can reject medical treatment.

The concept of autonomy or self-determination solely by the patient (even if competent) does not apply with equal force in all cultures. It is much less in the eastern cultures like the Japanese. There is social, economic and political community. There is greater acceptance of the sharing principle. Medicine in Japanese tradition is a humanitarian art, based on "sokuin" (sympathy, benevolence). It is influenced by Confucian thought and Buddhism.

The Jewish tradition also gives priority to beneficence, when it conflicts with autonomy. The precedence of beneficence over autonomy may not be upheld by law but it has the sanction of tradition.

Discharge Against Medical Advice

One of the problems a doctor faces occasionally in a healthcare institution is when a patient may not want to continue the treatment and may want to leave the hospital against medical advice. The doctors and other health care professionals may feel frustrated. But the patient has the right to leave at his/her will. It is best to get a signed statement from the patient (or the guardian in the case of a minor or incompetent person). But, the patient cannot be forced to sign. The doctor must warn the patient (and guardian) as patiently and carefully as possible of the need to continue the treatment. If the patient still insists on leaving, he/she has the right to leave. It must be so documented.

Palani, a 12-year-old boy, was admitted for fever of unknown origin. He had been in the hospital for 7 days. The hospital was giving free treatment. But the parents wanted him to be discharged. Their explanation was:

i. The diagnosis has been taking too long. The fever was still persisting.
ii. The parents were daily workers. They had to leave their work to find time to visit their child.
iii. They had to spend money for transport and other expenses.

The doctor was unhappy. He had been trying his best. He did not want the patient to be discharged till a proper diagnosis was made and specific treatment instituted. The doctor tried to explain the situation but the parents were insistent.

The patients (and the parents/guardians in the case of minors/incompetent persons) have the right to determine whether they want to continue with the treatment.

There can be a few exceptions of a life-threatening nature.

INFORMED CONSENT

'Consent' did not feature as a central part of doctor-patient relationship until recent times. There is no reference to this concept in Indian or Greek Medicine. The patient seeks the help of the doctor and there is a position of trust, as the doctor was pledged to 'beneficence' and 'non-maleficence'.

The notion of consent is an attempt to safeguard patient's autonomy. It acquired momentum in parallel with the ideas of individual liberty and freedom of choice.

What do Patients Want?

- Honest, unbiased, up-to-date information about their illness.
- The likely outcome.
- The benefits and risks of different interventions.
- Help to identify and secure their treatment preferences.
- Advice supported by the best available evidence.

Doctor's Opinion

- Informed consent breeds suspicion and mistrust.
- Patients want doctors to take responsibility.
- Patients do not understand the emphasis on consent forms.
- Patients have full faith in the knowledge, skills and conpetence of the doctor.
- 'Doctor knows best'.
- 'Informed consent' erodes the doctor-patient relationship.

Patients become anxious and distressed when the problem is discussed openly and frankly.

- Can the information be shared during an emergency?
- Can patients respond appropriately during a crisis?
- Getting informed consent is a needless nuisance.
- It is difficult to explain the procedures to the patient.

Informed consent has become a central issue in medical ethics today.

- A person's right to be fully aware of the extent, course and implications of his/her medical condition.
- Patient's right to participate in and influence the medical actions that may be undertaken or withheld.

The patient has the right to decide what shall be done to him or her. Consent is necessary. This consent respects the patient's right to self-determination. It must be "informed consent". It has evolved as an essential component of doctor-patient relationship.

Does 'informed consent' provide a defence for doctors against legal liabilities? Sections 87-93 of IPC deal with consent to procedures on the person. Section 87 permits a patient above 18 years to give consent to suffer harm by a doer where the harm is not done with the intention to cause death or grievous hurt. Section 88 absolves the doctor (doer) who may cause harm (without intention to cause death) from charges of committing offence, provided it is done for the person's benefit and in good faith. Section 90 says that if consent is given under fear of injury or under a misconception, it is not a consent.

Incomplete information is a misconception of omission.

The qualified doctor knows best the scientific consequences of any particular intervention. The patient has to live through the consequences of the intervention. Every person holds a set of constantly updated values, specific to that individual. These serve to guide decision-making.

A doctor has a duty to a patient to give adequate facts necessary to form an informed consent to the proposed procedure. There arises a "therapeutic partnership".

Many questions arise:

- What information should be given and when?
- Who else (other than the patient) should be involved in the information?
- Are there situations where the information should be kept away from the patient?
- How should consent be obtained? How should it be recorded?
- If the patient is under mental stress (as happens in all serious illness), is the consent valid?
- Who can give consent on behalf of minors/mentally incompetent?

When recommending a particular line of treatment or management, the doctor must provide the patient with all necessary information. The information must be:

- truthful
- adequate
- given tactfully, at the right time and in appropriate style and language.

The information must give the benefits and risks of the proposed line of management and the alternatives available with their benefits and risks.

It is not enough if information is given. Ensure that the patient comprehends it. Communication requires that the recipient understands the information without distortion. A number of questions arise:

- How can comprehension by the patient (and/or relatives) be assured?
- How does the doctor deal with patients of limited intelligence and from different cultural and linguistic backgrounds?
- Is it possible to communicate effectively medical information such that the patient comprehends it?
- How do we determine that the information given is adequate?
- Can there be a situation such that there is information overload, confusing the patient?

It is the duty of the doctor to make all reasonable efforts to ensure comprehension. If that is done and then the patient gives the consent, we have "informed consent". It is the willing and uncoerced acceptance of the proposed medical intervention. It is the acceptance of the intervention with its risks and benefits after considering the alternatives available.

The moral and legal obligations of disclosure by the doctor varies with the situation. In an emergency situation, the amount of information to be provided will not be much. Precious time must be saved. The benefits of the intervention will far outweigh the risks. In the case of elective procedures (non-life-threatening), much more information has to be provided. The need for adequate information is still more in the case of experimental procedures.

It is common thinking that it is extremely difficult, if not impossible, to get 'informed consent' from most of the people in India because of illiteracy. Will the patient be able to make a reasoned choice from among the alternatives available? Can they appreciate the differences? It has been found from studies that decision-making did not depend on the educational level or the socioeconomic situation. It is dependent on the adequacy of information.

Can a doctor advance the plea for not carrying out an indicated procedure in a life-saving situation, that 'consent' was not given by the patient? An interesting case occurred in the State of Kerala. A patient with acute abdominal pain was admitted to a Government Hospital. The duty doctor (a surgeon) diagnosed the condition as perforated appendix with peritonitis. It required an immediate operation. But the operation was not performed by the surgeon. The patient died the next day. The relatives sued the doctor and the Government for damages.

In the defence, the doctor stated that he could not carry out the operation because the patient did not give consent. This had not been documented. The court rejected the plea and awarded damages against the doctor.

The case went to the High Court on appeal. Two surgeons were called as expert witnesses. They stated that they would have operated unhesitatingly on the patient even without explicit consent.

The Kerala High Court upheld the decision of the lower court. The High Court observed that, when a doctor advances the plea that the patient did not give the consent, the burden is on the doctor to prove that the operation or treatment was not carried out because of the refusal of the patient to give the consent. It is more so in life-threatening situations. The patient had submitted himself to the doctor for treatment. There was implicit consent. The refusal of consent must be made out by the person alleging it.

A doctor is the best judge to decide whether or not an operation is necessary when a patient is brought to him. If an operation is a must to save the patient and it cannot wait, the operation must be performed with the implied consent of the patient.

Q. Is explicit consent necessary from a patient in critical condition but in full possession of his or her senses, before undertaking any procedure on him or her?
The decision of the court and the general consensus have been that the formality of an express consent from the patient must be dispensed with, considering the critical condition and urgency for operation. The high court also relied on the evidence of other surgeons. The accepted practice is also important. If the patient opposes the proposed procedure, it must be documented. The person alleging that there was refusal must establish it.

Q. If by the doctor's refusal to undertake the surgery the patient later dies, what is the liability of the doctor? If after the operation, the patient dies, what is the liability?

The court has held that the doctor is liable, unless the doctor could establish that

1. the operation was not indicated and the practice is not to operate under the given situation of the patient's condition, facilities available, etc., or
2. the patient refused the operation and it is so documented. The patient being in critical condition, the operation is bound to be risky and the patient may die. Section 88 of the Indian Penal Code gives complete protection to the doctor.

It is known that the operation might be followed by death. If the operation is carried out in good faith and not intending to cause death but with the intention of giving the benefit of the urgently required operation and with competence, the doctor is not liable. There is no criminal liability. There is also no civil liability, if there is no negligence.

It is interesting to note the ancient teaching in such a situation. Charaka's advice is for the doctor to take into confidence the close relatives, the elders in the community and even state officials (equivalent to a court order) before undertaking procedures which might end in the death of the patient. The doctor is then to proceed with the risky but necessary treatment.

The situation of the patient quoted gives an example of where the doctor's responsibility to help the patient seems to over-ride the patient's freedom to choose. Such situations arise when

- the benefits are high,
- the risks of non-treatment are high, and
- the patient has somehow failed to understand the nature of his/her condition and the benefits and risks.

In such a situation what should the doctor do? Talk further with the patient and persuade (not coerce) the patient. If possible, get the opinion of a second doctor who could then talk to the patient. If everything fails, a legal authorization may be obtained or the refusal documented.

Sometimes, parents of children may refuse consent for particular procedures (like blood transfusion) on children on religious or other grounds. The decision, at least in USA, has been "parents may make martyrs of themselves but they are not free to make martyrs of their children". It may be best to get a court decree.

There can be many difficulties in getting 'informed consent'. Information can create anxiety. Sometimes, patients may not want to know the true situation. In some situations, we give placebos. The patient is in the dark regarding the nature of intervention. Placebos are justified in certain conditions:

- Those which have a known high response rate of placebo, e.g. mild mental depression.
- Alternative is the use of a drug with known toxicity or addiction, e.g. morphine, in the case of postoperative pain.
- Patient insists on some medication.

Competence to Consent

Consent is the informed exercise of a choice which entails an opportunity to evaluate knowledgeably the options available and the risks attended on each.

"A person is competent for the task of giving a free and informed consent if:

1. she is generally informable and cognitively capable of performing the actions involved in making a decision;
2. she knows that decision-making requires these tasks;
3. she knows how to perform these tasks; and
4. given the situation, we can reasonably expect her to be able to make decisions".

—White, Beeky Cox: Competence to consent, Washington DC, Georgetown University Press, 1994, p. 209.

Competence does not disappear just because professional decisions are contested nor does compliance guarantee its presence.

Consent by Proxy

Can anyone else, e.g. a family member, consent on behalf of the patient? Legally, they can do so only if they are authorised by the court to be the guardian of the patient. But often we get the consent of close relations. The members of the family do not have the legal authority to make crucial decisions on behalf of adult patients, unless there is a court order to that effect. But there is a moral authority. The close family members can be expected to help the patient and to make decisions in the "best interests" of the patient.

Consent by Minors

If the medical problem is not an emergency, minors can be treated only with the consent of their parents. There are exceptions. Minors living away from parents, e.g. students in hostels and colleges, cannot be expected to get parental consent, before being treated. In USA, minors indulging in drug abuse, having venereal diseases or suffering from mental illness can be treated without the consent of parents.

CHAPTER 7

Rights of Patients

A patient is a person. Every person, whether well or ill, has the right to be treated with human dignity.

A patient is a person with a unique problem. A patient is a person who is suffering and needs help. It is necessary to recognize his/her rights. These rights are equal to those of anyone else in health. Prayer of the ancient physician Maimonides: "May I never see in the patient anything else but a fellow creature in pain".

Health being a basic necessity, the patient has the right to call for help. The Jewish tradition requires the physician to respond positively to the call of the patient for help. In fact, it obligates every individual to come to the help of a fellow human being. A physician who does not respond to the sick patient's call is regarded as one "who spills blood". "Neither shall thou stand idly by the blood of thy fellow". Just as it is obligatory for the physician to render care, it is mandatory for the patient to seek care.

Similar requirements are seen in other traditions and practices.

A PATIENT'S BILL OF RIGHTS

1. A patient has the right to considerate and respectful care.
2. The patient has the right to obtain from his physician complete current information concerning his diagnosis, treatment, and prognosis in terms the patient can be reasonably expected to understand.

   When it is not medically advisable to give such information to the patient, the information should be made available to an appropriate person in his behalf. He has the right to know, by name, the physician responsible for coordinating his care.
3. The patient has the right to receive from the physician information necessary to give informed consent prior to the start

of any procedure and/or treatment. Except in emergencies, such information for informed consent should include, but not necessarily be limited to the specific procedure and/or treatment, the medically significant risks involved, and the probable duration of incapacitation.

Where medically significant alternatives for care and treatment exist, or when the patient requests information concerning medical alternatives, the patient has the right to such information. The patient also has the right to know the name of the person responsible for the procedures or treatment.

4. The patient has the right to refuse treatment to the extent permitted by law and to be informed of the medical consequences of his action.
5. The patient has the right to every consideration of his privacy concerning his own medical care programme. Case discussion, consultation, examination and treatment are confidential and should be conducted discreetly. Those not directly involved in his care must have the permission of the patient to be present.
6. The patient has the right to expect that all communications and records pertaining to his case should be treated as confidential.
7. The patient has the right to expect that within its capacity a hospital must make reasonable response to the request of the patient for services. The hospital must provide evaluation, service, and/or referral as indicated by the urgency of the case.

   When medically permissible, a patient may be transferred to another facility only after he has received complete information and explanation concerning the need for and the alternatives to such a transfer. The institution to which the patient is to be transferred must first have accepted the patient for transfer.
8. The patient has the right to obtain information as to any relationship of his hospital to other health care and educational institutions in so far as his care is concerned. The patient has the right to obtain information as to the existence of any professional relationships among individuals, by name, who are treating him.

9. The patient has the right to be advised if the hospital proposes to engage in or perform human experimentation affecting his care or treatment. The patient has the right to refuse to participate in such research or projects.
10. The patient has the right to expect reasonable continuity of care. He has the right to know in advance what appointment times and physicians are available and where. The patient has the right to expect that the hospital will provide a mechanism whereby he is informed by his physician or a delegate of the physician of the patient's continuing health care requirements following discharge.
11. The patient has the right to examine and receive an explanation of his bill regardless of the source of payment.
12. The patient has the right to know what hospital rules and regulations apply to his conduct as a patient.

No catalogue of rights can guarantee for the patient the kind of treatment he has the right to expect. A hospital has many functions to perform including the prevention and treatment of diseases, the education of both health professional and patients, and the conduct of clinical research.

All these activities must be conducted with an overriding concern for the patient, and above all, the recognition of his/her dignity as a human being. Success in achieving this recognition assures success in the defence of the rights of the patient.

RIGHT OF ACCESS TO RECORDS

The sick person is most interested in his ailment. Can he/she see his/her medical records?

A patient can call for his/her medical records through the court. Till recently, it was considered that the patient did not have a right to his/her medical records. A recent judgement of the Bombay High Court has stated that the patient can ask for and get a copy of his/her own medical records. The Medical Council of India in its recent regulations has stated: "If any request is made for medical records either by the patients/authorized attendant or legal authorities involved, the same may be acknowledged and documents shall be issued within the period of 72 hours".

Other countries have legislation which gives a statutory right to the patient to obtain access to their health records. The Access to Health Records Act, 1990 confers the right subject to some important exceptions.

There are people who advocate giving access and others opposing it. Points in favor:

1. it would result in greater accuracy in record keeping,
2. it enhances trust and removes suspicion, and
3. the patient has an inherent right to records about him.

Points against:

1. it can seriously undermine the relationship between doctor and patient, and
2. patient's own interpretation of the notes can be faulty.

There are exceptions to the right of access to records:

- Where, in the doctor's opinion, information was likely to cause serious harm to the physical or mental health of the patient or any other individual.
- Where information relates to or is provided by an individual other than the patient or by another healthcare professional, if that individual can be identified or withholds consent.

One of the problems of free access to medical records is the possibility of developing defensive attitude to record writing and even treatment, because of the possibility of future litigation. But the overall view is to make the records available to the patient (guardian/parent, in the case of incompetent person/child). Care must be exercised to ensure that the records are not available to others.

CHAPTER 8

Irrational Drug Therapy

Drugs are important in:
- *prevention* of diseases (e.g. vaccines, vitamin A),
- *cure of disease* (e.g. antibiotics in infections, antidotes in poisoning),
- *alleviation of symptoms* (e.g. analgesics in pain, oral rehydration salts in diarrheas), and
- *rehabilitation* (in some of the physical and mental illnesses and disabilities).

Modern drugs are powerful. They are highly beneficial, if used with skill and caution. But considerable harm can be done if the drugs are used irrationally. Such irrational use is unethical.

> "The physician who sets about to treat a disease, without knowing anything about it, is to be punished even if he is a qualified physician; if he does not give proper treatment, he is to be punished more severely; and if by his treatment, the vital functions of the patient are impaired, he must be punished most severely".
>
> —Kautilya Arthasastra

WHAT IS RATIONAL DRUG THERAPY?

It is the prescribing and use of the right drugs, in the right doses, at the right time and for the right duration in individual with the right diagnosis and indication.

Rational drugs have scientifically proven clinical efficacy with favorable benefit: Risk ratio. They are of adequate quality and are cost-effective.

Efficacy

Efficacy is defined as the ability of the drug to produce the intended (preventive/curative/symptomatic) effect. The outcome is favorable when used in the correct manner.

Benefit: Risk Ratio

This gives the efficacy and safety as opposed to undesired effects and misuse potential. This concept can be used for a single drug or for comparison between two or more drugs.

Quality

The quality of the drug reaching the consumer must be assured. Quality assurance must satisfy:

- *Identity*: The correct ingredients must be present;
- *Potency*: The ingredients must be present in the correct quantities;
- *Purity*: Drugs should not have contaminants, chemical or bacterial;
- *Bioavailability*: Rate and extent of absorption into the bloodstream and tissues must give the intended effect.

In India, there are about 20,000 manufacturers (large, medium, small and tiny) of whom over 3,000 are loan licensees. The loan licensees produce drugs for the larger producers (multinational or national) and the drugs are then marketed by the larger firms. The Government had announced the abolition of loan licences. The powerful pharmaceutical lobby was up in arms against the Government decision and hence, the decision was not implemented.

Irrationality in Drug Use

This arises out of irrational:

- drug production, marketing and availability,
- prescribing habits, or
- use by the consumer.

It is necessary to eliminate the production, marketing and availability of irrational drugs. As long as irrational drugs continue to be produced and marketed, they are likely to be used. It is therefore essential to weed out all:

- hazardous drugs (with unfavorable benefit: risk ratio), and
- useless drugs (not effective).

Such drugs should not be allowed to be produced or imported. A number of drugs and combinations of drugs have been banned in our country. Some of the manufacturers have obtained stay orders from courts. These drugs were banned on the basis of the recommendations of the Drugs Consultative Committee and the Drugs Technical Advisory Board. There is no reason to use these drugs when the experts have decided that they should not be used. Some drugs banned in other countries are available in our country. It is not advisable to use them.

DRUG PROMOTION

Drugs are promoted by various means. It is necessary that the WHO guidelines are followed in the promotion of drugs. Drug Promotion (adapted from "Ethical criteria for medicinal drug promotion", WHO, Geneva, 1988 and modified later).

1. Promotional practices related to medicinal drugs should be in keeping with acceptable, ethical standards and consistent with the search for truthfulness and righteousness. They apply to any product promoted as medicine. Active promotion within a country should take place only with respect to drugs legally available in the country.
2. Promotion should be in keeping with national health policies and in compliance with national regulations.
3. a. All promotion-making claims concerning medicinal drugs should be:
   reliable,
   accurate,
   truthful,
   informative,
   balanced,
   up-to-date,
   capable of substantiation, and
   in good taste.

   b. They *should* not contain misleading or unverifiable statements, have *omissions* likely to induce medically unjustifiable drug use, or give rise to undue risks.

   c. The word "safe" should only be used if properly qualified.

   d. Comparison of products should be factual, fair and capable of substantiation.

e. Promotional material should not be designed so as to disguise its real nature.

4. Scientific data in the public domain should be made available to prescribers and any other person entitled to receive it on request, as appropriate to their requirements.
5. Promotion in the form of *financial or material benefits* should not be offered to or sought by healthcare practitioners to influence them in the prescription of drugs.
6. Scientific and educational activities should not be deliberately used for promotional purposes.
7. The wording and illustrations in advertisements to physicians and related health professionals should be fully consistent with the approved scientific datasheet for the drug concerned or other source of information with similar content. The text should be fully legible.
8. Information that promotional advertisement should contain:
   - the name(s) of the active ingredient(s) using either international non-proprietary names or the approved generic name of the drug;
   - the brand name, if used;
   - content of active ingredient(s) per dosage form or regimen;
   - name of other ingredients known to cause problems;
   - approved therapeutic uses;
   - dosage form or regimen;
   - side effects and major adverse drug reaction;
   - precautions, contra indications and warnings;
   - major interactions with other drugs;
   - name and address of manufacturer or distributor;
   - reference to scientific literature as appropriate.
9. Advertisements to the general public should help people to make rational decisions on the use of drugs determined to be *legally available* without a prescription. While they should take account of people's legitimate desire for information regarding their health, they should not take undue advantage of people's concern for their health. They should not generally be permitted for prescription drugs or to promote drugs for certain serious conditions that can be treated only by qualified health practitioners.
10. To fight drug addiction and dependency, scheduled narcotic and psychotropic drugs *should not be* advertised to the general public.
11. While health education aimed at children is highly desirable, drug advertisements *should not be* directed at children.

12. Advertisements may claim that a drug can cure, prevent, or relieve an ailment *only* if this can be substantiated. They should also indicate, where applicable, appropriate *limitations* to the use of the drug.
13. When lay language is used, the information should be consistent with the approved scientific data sheet or other legally determined scientific basis for approval. Language which brings about *fear or distress* should not be used.
14. Information on price to the consumer shoud be accurately and honestly portrayed.
15. Medical representatives should make available to prescribers and dispensers *complete* and unbiased information for each product discussed, such as an approved scientific data sheet or other source of information with similar content.
16. Medical representatives *should not* offer inducements to prescribers and dispensers. Prescribers should not *solicit* such inducements. In order to avoid over promotion, the main part of the remuneration of medical representatives should not be directly related to the volume of sales they generate.
17. Post-marketing scientific studies and surveillance *should not be* misused as a disguised form of promotion.

IRRATIONAL PRESCRIBING

Prescribing can be irrational under a variety of conditions:

1. Unnecessary prescribing: There may be no true indication for a drug. Before prescribing a drug, consider:
   - Is a drug necessary? Non-drug therapy may be more beneficial.
   - Will this drug help in correcting the disorder?

   Drugs are often used as substitutes for caring.
2. Extravagant prescribing: Is this drug unnecessarily too costly? Can a less costly but equally effective (in the given situation) drug be used? Is the patient made to pay more because of the brand name? The brand names and patents increase the cost.

> "My idea of a better ordered world is one in which medical discoveries would be free of patents and there would be no profiteering from life or death"
>
> —Smt Indira Gandhi
> at the World Health Assembly (1981)

Cost-effectiveness is often lost sight of. Unnecessarily high cost may be due to various factors including costly packaging. When considering the cost, take into account the cost of total treatment.

3. Overprescribing: There is a tendency to prescribe too much of the drug—too large dose or for too long.
4. Underprescribing: Occasionally the needed drug is not prescribed or the dosage is too small or the length of treatment is too short.
5. Incorrect prescribing: The diagnosis may not be correct and, hence the wrong drug may be prescribed. Ask the question: Is this the right drug? Have I selected the best agent available? the best formulation and best route of administration?

   Adjustments have to be made for age (child or elderly) or for other coexisting problems like hepatic damage or renal insufficiency. Certain drugs may be contraindicated in pregnancy.
6. Multiple prescribing: Too many drugs may be prescribed. This may be due to inability to form a correct diagnosis or other cause. Possibilities of drug interactions increase with polypharmacy.

Patient Information

The doctor must ensure that the patient (or some one on behalf of the patient, especially in the case of the incompetent patient) gets good, reliable information about the use of the drug:

- Name of the drug.
- How much to take, when, how often, and any relationship to food.
- The likely side effects, special precautions and toxic effect.
- Action to be taken if there are adverse effects.
- What to do if the expected results are not seen?

DRUG LEGISLATION FOR RATIONAL DRUG POLICY

There are a number of laws passed at different times governing the production, marketing, prescribing and use of drugs.

The Drugs and Cosmetics Act, 1940

This Act was enacted to prevent substandards in drugs. The Act prohibits the import and manufacture of misbranded, adulterated or spurious drugs. The Act did not have any provision to prohibit irrational or hazardous drugs. A new section was added in 1982. Section 26 A reads: "If the Central Government is satisfied that the use of any drug or cosmetic is likely to involve any risk to human beings or animals or that any drug does not have the therapeutic value claimed or purported to be claimed for it or contains ingredients and in such quantity for which there is no therapeutic justification and that in the public interest it is necessary or expedient so to do, then, the Government may, by notification in the official Gazette, prohibit the manufacture, sale or distribution of such drug or cosmetic".

The Drugs and Magic Remedies (Objectionable Advertisement) Act, 1954

The Act aims "to control the advertisement of drugs in certain cases, to prohibit the advertisement for certain purposes of remedies alleged to possess magic qualities". The Act lists in the schedule certain diseases or disorders. The idea seems to be to prevent lay persons being carried away by misleading advertisements.

DRUGS UNDER SPECIAL CIRCUMSTANCES

Special care must be exercised when prescribing drugs in certain situations.

Children

Children differ from adults in the response to drugs. The risk of toxicity is greater because of:
- deficient metabolic processes,
- inefficient renal clearance,
- different organ sensitivities, and
- inadequate detoxifying systems.

Prescriptions must always give the age of the child.

Elderly

Many conditions are psychosomatic. Drugs are a poor remedy. Often, to relieve the symptoms, multiple drugs are given. They may produce interactions.

In old age, the absorption, metabolism and excretion of drugs are altered. Patient compliance may be poor. There may be confusion. Instructions must be clear, simple and explicit.

Pregnancy

Avoid, if possible, all drugs during pregnancy. This is especially so in the first trimester. Some drugs are absolutely contraindicated.

Breastfeeding

Only essential drugs which cannot be avoided should be given to a nursing mother. Drugs may cause toxic reactions in the infant.

Disease of Liver

Drugs must be administered with caution in persons with liver disease. Keep the drugs to the minimum.

Diseases of Kidney

If excretion of the drug or its metabolic products by the kidney is reduced, toxicity may be produced. Avoid nephrotoxic drugs to the extent possible. The dose must be monitored carefully in each individual patient.

> "Doctors pour drugs of which they know little, to cure diseases of which they know less, into patients of whom they know nothing"
>
> —Voltaire
>
> Should we not change it?

CHAPTER 9

Right to Life

The Universal Declaration of Human Rights, article 3 says: "Everyone has the right to life, liberty and security of person". Article 6 of the International Covenant on Civil and Political Rights says: "Every human being has the inherent right to life". According to these and other declarations, right to life is inherent in a person, a human being.

Who is a human being? Who is a person? When does a developing embryo become a person? Different people interpret personhood differently. It is extremely difficult to draw a line and say that the developing zygote or fetus becomes a person from a particular time. Development takes place all the time. The fertilized ovum has within it all the components needed for growth and development into the full person.

Damages are claimed if an injury is caused to the fetus in the womb. It would mean that the fetus is a person. Can the life of that person be ended by procedures approved by others?

Some people have interpreted that the developing fetus can be considered a person, when the fetus is viable and capable of independent existence if removed from the milieu of the uterus. This period is progressively being reduced due to advances in medicine. Others have stated that the developing embryo can be considered a person when the brain starts developing, drawing the analogy of brain death. Still others think that it should be the stage when there is no longer the possibility of 'twinning'. According to them the question of uniqueness of the person can come only when there is possibility of development of one person only and not when two persons can develop. Most of the people agree that personhood comes on when fertilization occurs. There is no separation from one stage to another. It is a continuum.

ABORTION

Abortion is an issue which has people against it under any circumstances, for it under almost all circumstances, or for it under certain defined circumstances. Some people are neutral.

Indian law allows abortion. The Medical Termination of Pregnancy Act, 1971, says that pregnancy can be terminated if:

i. the continuance of the pregnancy would involve a risk to the life of the pregnant woman or of grave injury to her physical or mental health; or
ii. there is substantial risk that if the child were born, it would suffer from such physical or mental abnormalities as to be seriously handicapped.

There are explanations as to what would cause a grave injury.

Taking all into consideration, there are a number of possible categories of indications when termination of pregnancy is legal:

Therapeutic: When the physical or mental health of the person (mother) is likely to be at risk by carrying the pregnancy to term.

Eugenic: When the pregnancy is likely to result in the birth of a seriously handicapped child.

Personal: When the pregnancy has occurred inspite of using accepted methods of contraception or is alleged to have resulted from rape.

The categories would include almost every case where the couple desire abortion. It is, in effect, abortion on demand.

Abortion used to be practised clandestinely before the Act and, most often, by unqualified person. This resulted often in death or sepsis, with its attendant complications. The passing of the Act made medical termination of pregnancy legal (and by qualified persons in an approved set-up). Still, illegal abortion continues.

The codes of conduct and various declarations are opposed to this termination of pregnancy. The Declaration of Geneva (adopted by the World Medical Association at Geneva, 1948) says:

"I will maintain the utmost respect for human life, from the time of conception".

Termination of pregnancy brings out conflicts between the rights of two persons: The rights of the mother and the rights of the child in the womb. Has the mother the right to have the child in the womb destroyed? Does not the unborn child have the right to life? Has the doctor the right to kill the child in the womb at the request of the mother?

In traditional societies, the decision to abort is often taken not by the mother but by elders in the family. The mother may be forced to do something which she may not want to do. In other instances, the pregnant woman may herself request an abortion. Sometimes, the mother feels guilty about the termination of the life of the child and may have deep regret over the abortion done. Give time for reflection over the contemplated action. The doctor should discuss the matter with the mother and others concerned (the father of the child, elders in the family) and also suggest possible options. The choice of the mother to have an abortion done may be due to:

- possible disruption of academic career,
- need to give up a job (affecting success in career), or
- anticipated social disgrace in having an illegitimate child.

In almost all such instances, calm reflection can lead to avoidance of abortion. The mother herself may want to rear the child or may give the child for adoption.

> "An intrauterine fetus was noted to have moderate hydrocephalus with an unimpressive cerebral mantle thickness. Junior colleagues suggested an elective termination of pregnancy. However, the couple wished to continue to term. The child was delivered and underwent a shunt surgery. The child was then lost to follow-up. Last week on a cheerful, sunny morning, in walked a five-year bubbly, bright boy with his proud parents. He had surpassed his classmates in IQ tests and was a consistent topper. This promising brilliance was the same hydrocephalic fetus who at one stage was being denied entrance into this world".
>
> —The Indian Journal of Medical Education, 34(1):31-35, 1995.

CHAPTER 10 Sex Preselection and Female Feticide

INTRODUCTION

The Indian Society, like many other societies, is pro-male. A son is expected to support his parents in old age. Thus a son is an old age security. In the patriarchal system, the son continues the family lineage. According to the Hindu religious custom, the son has to perform certain rites on the death of the parents. Female babies can mean dowry at marriage and, therefore, a burden for the family.

India is one of the few countries in the world where women are proportionately less in number than males. The sex ratio in India is 933 females to 1,000 males (Census 2001). What is worse is the child (0-6 years) sex ratio. There was a decline of 18 points in 2001 compared to the 1991 census figures. There was a decline in the sex ratio of 17 points in 1991 compared to 1981 census. This decline coincided with advent of sex determination tests and selective abortion of female fetuses.

Prenatal sex determination is most often carried out with the intention of rejecting the female fetus. If the test shows that it is a female fetus, an abortion is carried out by the doctor at the request of the parents. There are very many such abortion clinics. The public opinion is against it (when it comes to the individuals and the doctors, directly involved, the ethical issues are forgotten). There was a hue and cry.

Female Feticide

There is increasing concern over female feticide. While earlier, there was abortion irrespective of the sex of the fetus, in recent years, there is increased use (misuse) of technology (e.g. amniocentesis, ultrasound) to determine the sex of the unborn baby with the objective of aborting the fetus, if it is female. This had led to an intolerable situation of worsening the sex ratio, with disastrous consequences.

Census 2001

The sex ratio (females per 1,000 males) of the child population (0-6 age group) which was 945 in 1991 has fallen drastically to 927 in the 2001 census. A significant part of this fall has been attributed to female feticide. Doctors are involved in the prenatal diagnosis of sex and subsequent termination of pregnancy.

Responding to the demands raised, a new Act was passed by the Parliament.

Prenatal Diagnostic Techniques (Regulation and Prevention of Misuse) Act 1994 became the law of the country in 1996. The objective was to stop discrimination against the female sex. Prenatal sex determination followed by sex selective termination of pregnancy is a form of violence against women.

Sex Selection is Illegal, Immoral and Unethical

Sex selection is discriminatory. It is illegal, immoral and unethical. It is illegal because it is against the law. It is immoral because it denies equality of the sexes. It is unethical because it is against the ethical principles of beneficence, non-maleficence and justice. The right of the female to be born is denied.

Women are Demeaned

The practice of sex selection reinforces the current attitudes and practices which discriminate against girls and women. Women as a class are demeaned by the practice, which seeks to avoid the birth of the female child.

Sex Selection a Crime against Society

Sex selection and selective abortion of the female child is not only a crime against the individual, it is also a crime against society. Such practices exaggerate the already existing imbalances in the sex ratio, which will have adverse social effects. This has been seen in China, with the one-child norm and son preference.

Dowry and Other Social Evils

There are many arguments brought forward in support of the despicable practice of sex selection. The first is the practice of dowry. The answer to the problem of dowry is to attack the dowry system and not to kill the female child. We have to improve the status of women in our society.

Female Feticide and Female Infanticide

Another argument in favor of female feticide is that it is preferable to female infanticide. There cannot be comparisons; it is not a question of which evil is relatively more unethical. Female feticide and female infanticide are to be condemned equally.

Pre-natal Diagnostic Techniques

There are a number of prenatal diagnostic techniques (PNDT). The most frequently used method is ultrasound. It is non-invasive. The results are immediate. When performed by skilled operators, the sex can be determined to some extent of accuracy. The other methods are amniocentesis (lengthy time in getting results) and *chorionic villus* sampling (can be performed very early in gestation). There are other newer methods.

Supreme Court and Prenatal Diagnostic Techniques

Ultrasound is the most common method of misuse of the prenatal diagnostic techniques. The Supreme Court has taken cognizance of this fact. The court has directed the manufacturers of the ultrasound machines and the State Governments to get the names and addresses of the clinics/persons to whom the ultrasound machines had been sold. The states had been asked to ensure that these clinics are registered and they maintain proper records and do not violate the law.

What do the Medical Councils say?

"**2. The Physicians responsibility**

The honoured ideals of the medical profession imply that the responsibilities of the physician extend not only to individuals but also society (sex selection and female feticide affect the society).

9. Evasion of legal restrictions

"The physician will observe the laws of the country in regulating the practice of medicine and will not assist others to evade laws".

—Medical Council of India

The new Indian Medical Council (professional conduct, etiquette and ethcis) Regulations 2002 are more explicit:

"**1.9. Evasion of legal restrictions**

The physician shall observe the laws of the country in regulating the practice of medicine and shall also not assist others to evade such laws. He should be cooperative in observance and enforcement of sanitary laws and regulations in the interest of public health. A physician should observe the provisions of the State Acts like.... Prenatal Sex Determination Act, 1994....

7.6. On no account sex discrimination test shall be undertaken with the intent to terminate the life of a female fetus developing in her mother's womb, unless there are other absolute indicators for termination of pregnancy as specified in the Medical Termination of Pregnancy Act 1971. Any Act of termination of pregnancy of normal female foetus amounting to female foeticide shall be regarded as professional misconduct on the part of the physician leading to a penal erasure besides rendering him liable to criminal proceedings as per the provisions of the Act".

The Delhi Medical Council, 2001, has this to say:

"12.6 You should not advise, assist or conduct sex determination tests

12.7 You must not advise, assist in selective conception".

Other Methods of Sex Selection

There are other methods of sex selection. Sex selection can be preconception. This is done by separation of the spermatozoa with X and Y chromosomes. The success rate is said to be about 70%.

Preimplantation Genetic Diagnosis

Another method is by resorting to preimplantation genetic diagnosis, followed by implantation of the favored (male) embryo and selective destruction of the female embryo. The technique adds female embryocide to female feticide and female infanticide. The method is extremely expensive. There is need for an 'assisted reproduction unit'. The whims of the rich will be catered to. The not-so-rich will mortgage their homes and belongings in the pursuit of technology which could ultimately destroy the very fabric of the society.

Gen Select

There was an advertisement in the Times of India called 'Gen Select'. According to the advertisement, you can select the gender of the offspring. The technique is very costly. There is a pill and douche kit, nutriceuticals and dietary guidelines.

All these techniques are subject to the same ethical and legal objections as the prenatal diagnosis and selective termination of pregnancy.

Because of the loopholes in the Prenatal Diagnostic Techniques Act and the development of newer technologies for sex selection, a new bill has been passed by both Houses of Parliament (2002). It is awaiting the President's assent to become the law.

INFANTICIDE

There are some people who advocate the doing away of life of the newborn, if the newborn is defective. The defects (e.g. spina bifida) are compatible with life but may be a burden on the individual, the family and even the society. Such tendencies are seen more in the so-called developed countries. It is much less in India. Unfortunately, the number of people in favor of doing away with defective newborn is increasing with a change in value system.

Some people would advocate infanticide if it is a female child. In China, the proportion of newborn in 1979 was boys: 51.5%, girls: 48.5%. With the announcement by the Government of the one-child policy, the ratio changed drastically. In 1981, it became boys:58%, girls: 42%. Babies who die within 3 days of birth are considered stillborn and their births are not registered. Midwives are known to plunge a baby girl straight into a bucket of water at the moment of birth and record a stillbirth.

SEVERELY HANDICAPPED BABIES

Parents have the desire to have a child of a certain quality. A child with disability brings a burden for the family and the society.

Bringing up the child with disability can cost money and use up resources. But people cope up with the difficulties. In the bargain, the experience brings about better development of the people. There is a better appreciation of the higher values.

It is wrong to assume that making things easier will go to make happier people. Many people with disabilities achieve a very happy life, whereas apparently 'normal' people often lead a miserable life.

Babies are not able to consent to or refuse medical treatment to sustain life or allow its termination. Are the parents and doctors free to choose for the babies? Can death be a legally valid choice in the case of a severely disabled baby?

Babies are born with conditions, such as Down's syndrome or spina bifida. Can the parents together with the doctor decide whether the child with the disability should live or be allowed to die? If they can decide to do away with the life of the baby with disability (omit nutrition, surgery or other ordinary measures which would have been undertaken in a normal baby or resort to such procedures as would end the life), it would mean that the life of the child with disability is considered less valuable (so much less valuable that it is not worth preserving).

Ramani Kanakarajan, 36 years, is a stenographer. She had an amniocentesis which showed that her daughter *in utero* had Down's syndrome. "I had not planned to have any tests but had an amnio when the scan showed abnormality. When I got the result, I felt stunned. But it never occurred to me to have an abortion. I felt strongly that a child has been conceived and that child had a right to live". That child is now 4 years old. "My daughter is slow to learn but she is not really so different from normal children. She is lively, healthy and happy. She has brought us as much joy as our other three children".

Lawra Benedict, whose ten-year-old daughter Rita has Down's syndrome, has also found it an enriching experience. "I was only 28 when I had Rita. When I saw that she was Down's I was bitterly disappointed. I grieved for the perfect baby I had been expecting. But Rita is a darling. I love her. She tries so hard. I cannot describe the joy when she masters something. The handicap does not bother us. Rita is a child first and foremost".

CHAPTER 11

Assisted Reproductive Technologies

RESPONSE TO INFERTILITY

The desire to have a child is a basic human urge. Is the desire biological or social? Probably both factors operate. The innate desire (propagation of species?) is often driven by culture.

There are many social pressures to have children. Family and friends expect a couple to start a family, soon after marriage. There is a desire to have a heir who will inherit the property from the parents. Women were divorced in many societies because they failed to provide a heir. Often men resorted to a second marriage to get a heir.

In the Hindu culture, certain religious rites are performed by the son. There is also the deep seated feeling in almost all cultures that children are a blessing. Barren women are looked down upon by society. "The man without progeny is like a tree that yields no shade, which has no branches, which has no fruit and is devoid of any pleasing odor"—*Charaka Samhita.*

Chinese tradition also placed high value on having children. According to Mencius (next only to Confucius), not having a child isolates filial piety. He says: "Among the three vices which violated filial piety, the biggest one is being without offspring". Traditional Chinese believe that having no child is because of lack of virtue in the couple. There is heavy psychological pressure to extend the ancestor's life into future generations.

The realization that they cannot have children of their own can have damaging effects on the relationships of the couple.

Is infertility a disease needing medical treatment? It is not life-threatening nor does it lead to detectable bodily damage. Infertility is a malfunction. It is most often due to some disordered function, which calls for treatment. Many a time, no particular cause can be found, the rectification of which will lead to fertility.

Infertility can lead to psychological distress in those who are keen on having children. It can precipitate a mental disorder which can warrant treatment. In such instances, it would be better to treat the primary cause of infertility.

Infertility may be due to the male factor, female factor or due to both. In more than 30% of the couples, the abnormality is in the male. In about 20-25%, there is defective ovulation. 20% have problems involving the fallopian tube (often following pelvic inflammation). In about 25%, there is no apparent explanation for the infertility. Where infertility is due to defect in only one of the partners, should the other partner be denied the right to have a child?

ADOPTION

Adoption is not very popular in India, though it is very popular in the western countries. Many couples do derive considerable satisfaction from adoption. There is no dearth of babies available for adoption in our country (unlike western countries). There are many orphans and abandoned children waiting to be adopted. Many women who do not want to go through the pregnancy can be coaxed to continue the pregnancy and give birth to babies, instead of aborting them. This is especially so with single unmarried women. Such babies can be adopted even at the prenatal state. The desire to rear is satisfied.

RIGHT TO REPRODUCE

Is there a self-evident, natural right to reproduce? Natural law gives the freedom to reproduce. The individual can choose. It does not hold that it is necessary or even desirable that every individual should reproduce. Chastity is a respected value in most cultures and many follow it. The decision to beget a child belongs to the individual concerned. There should be no outside interference, unless there are good and valid reasons to the contrary. The infringement of the liberty must be for a justifiable cause.

Is there a Natural Right to Reproduce by Artificial Means?

If the main purpose of sexual intercourse is the conception and begetting of children, does it mean that not to assist infertile couples to reproduce is to deny a right and not fulfilling the purpose of the sex act? *A natural right is not to be provided by artificial means.* The freedom to reproduce does not mean that there is an obligation that the person should be helped to reproduce when the natural means fail.

Is there a right for single women to have a child by artificial insemination? There is an increasing demand in western countries. Section 13(5) of the Human Fertilisation and Embryology Act,1991 of UK states: "A woman shall not be provided with treatment services unless account has been taken of the welfare of any child which may be born as a result of the treatment (including the need of that child for a father)".

Begetting: There is a natural desire to beget. The individual wishes to have a child with a particular person, as an expression of their intimate relationship. In vitro fertilization with gametes from the two individuals can satisfy the desire. Gamete donation by another individual will not achieve it. The child is seen as an extension of self.

Bearing: When the couple is not able to conceive by natural means, and the defect is in the husband, artificial insemination by donor can overcome it and the mother can bear the child.

Rearing: The desire to rear children can be met by adoption. In surrogate motherhood, if the carrying mother provides not only her womb but also the ovum, the commissioning mother is enabled only to rear the child but not to beget or bear. The desire to rear a child can be a strong desire. In custody disputes between husband and wife, the issue most often is the desire to rear the child.

NEW TECHNOLOGIES OF REPRODUCTION

There has been a spurt of growth of newer technologies of reproduction. All of them raise ethical issues. They are expensive. They involve tests, hospitalization and number of trials until pregnancy is finally achieved.

Artificial Insemination

Artificial insemination may be by the husband (AIH) or by a donor (AID). In artificial insemination by husband, the offspring has the gametes from both parents. In artificial insemination by donor, the husband is not the real parent. It is necessary to get the consent of both parties before the procedure is carried out. The husband acquires legal rights and obligations as a natural father. The records must be kept confidential. They are not subject to inspection by anyone, except on court orders for good cause. Before carrying out the procedure, the doctor must explain that:

- there is no guarantee of pregnancy,
- there are possibilities of birth defects, and
- there are possibilities of transmitting diseases.

The doctor must then screen the donor adequately. There is a possibility that the doctor may be sued if the donor is not screened sufficiently for genetic defects and diseases or if the husband's consent is not obtained. In UK, screening for the potential transmission of human immunodeficiency virus is mandatory. The semen is kept frozen and the donor is tested again after 3 months to make sure that he does not show antibodies to HIV.

According to the Islamic point of view, artificial insemination may be done with the husband's semen but not that of another donor. It is only within the marriage contract that the progeny should be conceived. This applies to other assisted reproductive procedures also, like in vitro fertilization. Such technologies are permitted only between the husband and wife. The permissibility applies only as long as the marriage is valid.

In Vitro Fertilization

The ovum is fertilised and incubated outside the body (in the laboratory). The fertilized ovum (blastocyst) is then transferred to the uterus. In vitro fertilization and embryo transfer (IVF-ET) was originally undertaken in patients with infertility due to damaged, blocked or absent fallopian tubes. It was later extended to many other conditions of infertility and even where there are no anatomical abnormalities. IVF-ET may be resorted to in

- a married couple with a medical problem by which fertilization does not take place in the natural way, and
- a married couple without any medical problem.

More recently, the technique has been used in:

- single women, desiring a child, or
- homosexuals,

The first IVF-ET baby in India was born on August 6, 1986.

The Technique

- Induction of hyperovulation by hormones.
- Withdrawal of oocytes.

- Fertilization by spermatozoa. Cultivation *in vitro*.
- Transfer into the uterus.

In vitro fertilization may involve:

- extraction of oocytes from a woman, impregnation within the laboratory by her lawful husband's sperm;
- extraction of oocytes from a woman, fertilization in the laboratory with sperm provided by a person other than the husband;
- oocytes extracted from another woman and fertilized by the husband's sperm; or
- third parties provide both the oocytes and the sperm.

There are many ethical problems.

Both husband and wife must be freely consenting to in vitro fertilisation and embryo transfer.

There are always more ova fertilized, even after a number of them (3-4) have been placed in the uterus to ensure greater success (the success rate with even such multiple embryos is very small). What to do with the excess embryos? Who has the right to determine what to do with them? It is held that only the persons from whom the ovum and the sperms were obtained have the sole right to determine any future use to which the embryo may be put. If they do not agree or are deceased, the right passes on to the storage laboratory (?). To solve the problem of surplus of fertilizsed ova that are denied the opportunity of later replacement into the mother's uterus, some people advocate to limit the number of ova to be exposed to fertilization to that which would be replaced into the uterus, if all of them became fertilized. Only unfertilized ova are kept in cold storage. They can be used later, if necessary, until the desired pregnancy is achieved.

Since multiple embroys are used, there is the possibility of multiple births. There is also the possibility of premature births.

There is high-risk of abnormalities and defects in children produced by laboratory fertilization. There is responsibility of the doctor, who may be charged with medical and scientific negligence. Damages may be claimed by the couple. Can damages be claimed by the developing child? It has been held that, if doctors create life and exact a fee for their services, they should assume responsibility for ensuring that no disability will follow.

In IVF-ET, the consenting parents assume all responsibilities and the child gets all the rights and privileges of a lawful offspring.

Many ethical problems arise because after-all "test-tube babies are babies". There is need for control and legislation with respect to the embryo.

Recommendations of Warnock Committee, UK (The Lancet, July 28, 1984):

A new statutory licensing authority should be created. It should inspect all premises carrying out these procedures. The provision of artificial insemination by donor services without a licence for the purpose should be an offence.

Any unauthorized use of an in vitro embryo would in itself constitute a criminal offence.

No live human embryo derived from in vitro fertilization, whether frozen or unfrozen, may be kept alive, if not transferred to a woman, beyond fourteen days after fertilization, nor may it be used as a research subject beyond fourteen days after fertilization. The number of days was placed as fourteen because the primitive streak appears at 14 days in the embryo and establishes whether the embryo will develop into a single entity or twins, triplets or more.

Gamete Intrafallopian Transfer

The gamete intrafallopian transfer (GIFT) technique is used in cases of infertility unrelated to fallopian tube problems. It is used in conditions of failure of ovum release, ovum pick-up by the fimbria, impaired tubal sperm transport and other similar conditions. The ovary is stimulated to produce a large number of oocytes. They are 'harvested' by laparoscopic aspiration and inserted into the fallopian tube, along with washed spermatozoa. GIFT procedures bring the oocytes into direct contact with spermatozoa. India's first GIFT baby was born on January 6, 1988.

SIFT (Semen Intrafallopian Transfer) is a Variant of GIFT

The ethical issues are similar to those in IVF-ET.

Surrogacy

'Surrogate' means substitute. Surrogate motherhood means using the womb of another woman to obtain a child because the wife is unable or does not want to bear a child.

The Warnock Committee (UK) defined surrogacy as "the practice whereby one woman carries a child for another with the intention that the child should be handed over after birth". Surrogacy can be in different forms:

- The commissioning woman is the genetic mother, when she provides the ovum.
- The carrying woman is the genetic mother, when her ovum is fertilized.
- The genetic father is the husband of the commissioning woman.
- The genetic father may be an unknown donor.

Mother of Three Agrees to Bear German Couple's Baby

A few months ago, life looked rather bleak for Hansaben Patel; she had very little hope of getting out of the rut of a poverty stricken existence at Dhuma village, 15 km from Ahmedabad.

So when opportunity came in the form of a German couple, looking for a woman who could bear their child, Hansaben did not think twice before accepting. After all her dream of a better life for her children would become reality.

Johanna and Alejandro Perez were more or less at the end of their tether when they met Dr. Himanshu Bavishi and his wife Dr Falguni who run an in vitro fertilization (IVF) clinic in Ahmedabad. The German couple had just returned from a trip to the US where they had found surrogate mothers cost the earth.

Twenty nine-year-old Hansaben's role will be strictly that of a biological mother. The German couple's embryo developed by the IVF technique will be implanted in Hansaben's uterus. Genetically the baby will be 100% German and Hansaben will be paid ₹1 lakh for carrying the baby to term.

The Week, May 30, 1999

Surrogacy is resorted to:

- when the woman has a severe pelvic disease, not amenable to be remedied,
- when the woman has no uterus or has other congenital disorders, making the carrying of pregnancy impossible.

- where the woman had a condition making pregnancy medically undesirable, and
- where the woman does not want to undergo the inconvenience of carrying the baby in utero for the pursuit of career or for other reasons.

The arrangement is in the nature of a contract. But this contract is not valid. Either party may revoke it and then it cannot be enforced. The carrying woman may develop such great affinity to the child that she refuses to give up the child. The child might have congenital defects and other disorders; the commissioning couple may not accept the child. The carrying woman might have sexual relationship with other men and the child may be, or may be suspected to be, the result of such intercourse. The commissioning couple who expected to be genetic parents then refuses to take the child.

Sometimes, the surrogate mother may be a close relation (say, sister) of the commissioning couple. In other cases (most often), it is an outsider. Some payment is made to the carrying mother in consideration of the inconvenience, loss of employment and medical expenses. In addition, she may receive a very substantial sum for "inducement" and "difficulties" in carrying the child. This leads to commercialization (rent-a-womb). Bearing children for a financial consideration is to be condemned.

In surrogacy, the concept of the family faces difficulties. It threatens the institution of marriage, destroys maternal bonding, treats children as commodities and exploits poor women as vehicles to satisfy the whims and fancies of the rich. The subsequent transfer of parental responsibility is a form of adoption. The commissioning couple assume the parental responsibilities for the care of the child.

With respect to surrogacy for inconvenience, the Warnock Committee has this to say: "Surrogacy for inconvenience alone, i.e. where a woman is physically capable of bearing a child but does not wish to undergo pregnancy is totally ethically unacceptable. Even in compelling medical circumstances, the danger of exploitation of one human being by another appears to the majority of us to outweigh the potential benefit. That people should treat others as a means to their own ends, however desirable the consequences, must always be liable to moral objection. Such treatment of one person by another becomes positively exploitative when financial interests are involved".

There are many people who are totally against surrogacy, because the entire procedure is unethical. Even those who recommend the procedure wish to place legal restrictions. Because of large scale profits in arranging surrogacy, a number of agencies sprang up. The Warnock Committee recommended legislation to make it a criminal offence to set up or operate surrogate agencies, commercial or otherwise.

The various recommendations, after debate in the Parliament, were incorporated in the Surrogate Arrangements Act of 1985.

Surrogate mother has no genetic contribution to make.

Surrogacy is big business. It turns a normal biological function of a woman's body into a commercial contract. Surrogate services are advertised. Surrogates are recruited. Operating agencies make large profits. Surrogacy turns impoverished women into baby producers.

Some agencies insist that the surrogate must:

- be married and be a mother of atleast one healthy child;
- be medically and psychologically fit;
- abstain from cigarettes, alcohol and other drugs during pregnancy;
- agree to give up her parental rights after the baby is born.

The contracting couple adopts the baby soon after delivery, so that they become legal parents of the child.

RIGHTS OF CHILDREN

Apart from legal questions of legitamacy, some of the new technologies will produce children who do not know their genetic parents (one or both). It violates the right of the child to know his/her own genetic history. There are two choices when children are produced by donation of the gamete: Tell the truth or keep it a secret forever or till the child attains majority. In the case of artificial insemination by donor, anonymity is maintained.

ICMR GUIDELINES (PROPOSED)

A Committee constituted by the Indian Council of Medical Research (ICMR) and the National Academy of Medical Sciences has proposed guidelines for the regulation of clinics carrying out assisted reproductive procedures. The ICMR Director-General has stated that this had become necessary "as it was essentially a commercial venture with various spin-offs, such as assisting female feticide.

The code that the guidelines propose include:

- Sex selection at any stage of the fertilization procedure is not to be permitted.
- The clinic will obtain sperms only from a bank and not through a relative or known friend of either partners.
- Surrogacy would be considered only for patients for whom it would be physically or medically impossible to carry a baby to term.
- The embryos may be stored for five years if the couple agrees and used for other couples or for research.
- The sale or transfer of the human embryo or any part of it is prohibited. Human cloning should be banned.
- A child born through assisted conception would be presumed to have all rights of parentage, support and inheritance.
- An HIV-positive woman would not be refused such conception but counselled adequately about the possibility of transmission of the virus to the child".

—The Times of India, Bombay, 5 Sept., 2002.

CHAPTER 12 Care of the Terminally Ill

There comes a time in the care of the sick when it is assessed, as accurately as possible with the available means, that the patient is in a stage of terminal illness, with imminent death within a short period. Care and attention then will be focussed on support to make the remaining part of life as confortable as possible. With the increases in lifespan and more persons suffering from malignancies, the number of such persons requiring supportive care is increasing. More medical resources are being used for such persons. The doctor will be facing more and more problems of the aged and the care of the terminally ill.

The terminally ill may belong to various categories:

- those who are conscious or unconscious;
- those with or without artificial life support; and
- those who are severely incapacitated in different ways.

The conscious terminally ill patient may have intense pain. They need relief from pain. Other distressing symptoms, such as difficulty in breathing may be present. Relief is needed for these symptoms. Keeping them in comfort becomes an over-riding requirement.

DISCRETION: TO TELL OR NOT TO TELL

There is difference of opinion among doctors whether and how much to tell the patient, while caring for the terminally ill. A study carried out in the Postgraduate Institute of Medical Education and Research, Chandigarh, found that 69.2% of the doctors participating in the study believed in telling the truth to the patient; 30.8%

did not favor it. Those who favored telling the truth had a number of reasons for doing so:

- The patient can settle the family and other problems before death.
- The patient accepts death more peacefully. The patient prepares for the coming event.
- More effective palliative (especially pain reduction) treatment can be instituted, without worrying too much about the long-term effects of such treatment.
- The patient gets the opportunity to fulfill last wishes.
- It stops the patient and relatives from running round seeking treatment from different sources.
- Unnecessary and useless expenditure is curtailed.
- The patient has a right to know.

Those who were not in favor of telling the patient gave the following reasons:

- It frustrates and angers the patient.
- The family members' job of consoling the patient is made more difficult.
- It is difficult to tell the harsh truth.
- In desperation, the patient may turn to quackery.

However harsh and difficult, there is need to inform. The way the truth is told is important. It must be conveyed gradually and with compassion. There is need to train doctors in the art of sensitive communication. According to Charaka (*Charaka Samhita*, 600 BC) it should not be told bluntly; it might shock the patient. The patient must be told the truth tactfully. In the Indian situation, it would be wise to take into confidence the family members and close relations, in view of the family structure and close ties among relations.

When a patient becomes aware of the terminal nature of the illness, he/she passes through many stages. There is first a stage of denial: "It cannot happen to me". It is followed by anger: "Why should this happen to me". There is then a stage of "bargaining", in an attempt to gain more time. This is followed by a stage of depression and finally there is acceptance of the inevitable. All stages may not be seen in all patients. In the Indian situation, acceptance is often quicker.

Nearly all dying patients come to realize what is happening. There are a small number for whom telling the truth would be an act of needless cruelty. But the very large number value telling the truth.

Communicating Bad News

Communicating bad news (like diagnosis of cancer) is a very difficult task for the doctor. There is need for sensitivity, honesty and willingness to be available to the patient, as also strong patient-doctor relationship. Even when the news is given, it may not be registered/retained by the patient because:

- the language used (often too technical) may not be familiar to the patient;
- a single communication may be insufficient when the patient is in pain and is anxious of the outcome.

The doctor may resort to non-disclosure, full disclosure or individualised disclosure.

Non-disclosure

When there is fear and anxiety, the doctor may decide not to tell because the doctor thinks that:

- doctor knows what is best for the patient;
- the patient does not want to know; or
- the patient must be protected from bad news.

These assumptions are not valid. The competent patient has a right to know. He/she can then make choices. Most patients want to know the diagnosis. There may be short-term negative emotional impact, especially if the news is given abruptly; in the long-term, patients adjust well. Uncertainty about the diagnosis and future course of events is a major cause of distress. Disclosing the news often results in less anxiety and better overall adjustment. Even when not told directly by the doctor, most patients arrive at the conclusion, with information from other sources, the investigations and the treatment. Non-disclosure is untenable. It is a violation of the right to information. The patients and their relatives get an opportunity to decide on the future, when they have the right information. They can face death with courage and dignity.

Full Disclosure

Some doctors give full information (bad news) to every patient, as soon as the information becomes available. The doctor assumes that:

- the patients want to know the news, however bad it might be;
- the patient has the right to know the full information;

- the doctor has an obligation to give it; or
- the patient has to face the consequences and determine what is best for him/her.

It is true that the patient has the right to information; it is also true that the patient has the right not to receive the information, either in full or in part. There is need for freedom of choice. The timing is also important. The patient may be confused and anxious and may not be ready for the bad news. While most patients want to hear the truth about the diagnosis, prognosis and treatment, some do not want full disclosure or may not be ready for it.

Individualized Disclosure

Each patient is different and therefore, there is need to deal with the disclosure of information differently. The doctor assumes that:

- patients are different in their desire to know and their capacity to receive bad news;
- patients need time to absorb bad news;
- patient-doctor relationship is based on mutual trust and partnership in decision-making.

The amount of information given at any time and the actual timings are tailored to suit the individual patient and the situation. The doctor and patient determine the amount of information to be given/received. Patients are different in their capacity for assumption and coping with the bad news. There are dangers in breaking bad news abruptly. It can precipitate depression. There is need to build mutual trust which will encourage the patient to ask questions and remove doubts and misconceptions. The doctor and patient determine how much information the patient wants and is to be given as also how the information should be given, over what period of time. The patient would also determine who else can/should be present.

RELIEF OF PAIN

Historically, relief from pain has been a major goal of medicine. It improves the quality of life. In the case of the terminally ill, especially those with advanced malignancy, pain is a devastating symptom. Relief from pain is the most important need of the patient.

Many analgesics have important, undesirable side effects, such as respiratory depression. Hence, medication to relieve pain must be carried out skillfully. When larger doses are used, the side effects can be very marked. The respiratory depression may be such that death may be hastened. Will it be tantamount to active euthanasia?

It is essential to ensure that the remaining period of the patient's life is as pain-free as possible. The doctor has to be competent in pain therapy. There is the problem of double effect: Pain relief (desirable) and respiratory depression (undesirable). The intended effect is pain relief. The other effect is not intentional; it is secondary. If the primary aim is relief of pain and not to hasten death, even though the respiratory depression can be foreseen, it is ethically sound, provided all precautions are taken to use only the minimum drug necessary. If, on the other hand, the intention is to hasten death, thereby bringing relief of pain, the procedures will be ethically wrong. The morally objectionable effect (hastening death by respiratory depression) cannot be the means for the morally acceptable effect (relief of pain). At no time should the intention be to hasten death, though it might lead to it secondarily. The primary intention should be to relieve pain in the most competent manner. The dosages of medicines must be rational. What is necessary for relief of pain must be given and no more?

A 60-year-old lady, who had been operated upon for carcinoma of the breast developed bony metastases. There was intense pain. She was given morphine regularly. The morphine depressed her respiratory functions. Death was probably hastened.

The primary aim being relief of pain, the procedure was ethically acceptable.

Another factor to be considered is the level of consciousness. There is need to keep up meaningful communication with the members of the family, friends and others. Avoid clouding of consciousness to the extent possible. The aim of pain reducing medication should be to get optimum relief of pain with minimum diminution of consciousness. Further, relief of pain has many aspects; physiological, psychological, social and spiritual. All these factors must be considered and made use of. They could reduce the dosage of analgesics.

A patient nearing death has to consider his/her death and the effect of his/her death on others, especially the nearest and closest in the family. The treating doctor must try to help the patient in coping with these problems. With the breakdown of the joint family system, the care of the elderly has become the responsibility of medical -and social organizations. The doctor has a role to play. The doctor must also ensure that the spiritual needs of the patients, according to his or her faith, are also met.

There is very little point in withholding adequate medication for the relief of pain for fear of addiction to the drug. Addiction has no significance in terminally ill patients. It is irrational to withhold effective medicine, when death is likely to take place within a short period.

There have been many considered pronouncements on the need for giving relief. Lord Justice Devlin has said: "If the purpose of medicine.... restoration of health.... can no longer be achieved, there is still much for the doctor to do and he is entitled to do all that is proper and necessary to relieve pain and suffering even if the measures he takes may incidently shorten life". The philosopher Francis Bacon made this statement: "I esteem it the office of the physician not only to restore health but to mitigate pains and dolors, and not only when mitigation conduces to recovery but when it may serve to make a fair and easy passage".

It is difficult to face death. There is tendency for the doctor and the nurse to go away at the moment of death. But it is precisely at this time of breavement that the presence of the doctor and the nurse is needed.

EXTRAORDINARY MEANS OF PRESERVING LIFE

To what extent should efforts be made to preserve life in the case of the terminally ill? When there is no reasonable hope of benefit to the patient, there is no need to resort to extraordinary means or heroic measures to preserve life. Every decision to terminate specific treatment and not to resuscitate the terminally ill patient should be accompanied by efforts to provide maximum comfort to the patient. We have to continue all ordinary means, according to the circumstances of person, place, time and culture. There is the duty of doing good. All medicines, treatment, procedures and operations which offer a reasonable hope of achieving one or more goals of medical care are to be used. If they involve far too much expense or pain or excessive use of resources or excessive inconvenience to the patient and to others and does not give a reasonable hope of benefit to the patient, they would be extraordinary means. The doctor has no obligation to use such extraordinary means to prolong life (prolong death).

Ramanujam, a 69 years old, terminally ill patient, was being fed through a feeding tube. The patient wanted the feeding tube to be removed and all nutrition and hydration withdrawn. The family of the patient asked for the opinion of the doctor. Would it be ethical to comply with the request?

The care given could not be considered as extraordinary. It provided ordinary nutrition and fluids. It is also likely to make the patient more comfortable. The situation must be explained to the patient. The nutrition and hydration should be continued. What can be terminated are the specific medical measures against the particular disease and not the measures for the general well-being of the patient?

In USA, even artificial provision of nutrition and hydration have recently been considered as medical treatment; medical treatment can be rejected.

'Do not resuscitate' orders are very much in vogue in many western countries. There is a growing inclination among doctors to do the same in our country also, especially in the larger cities. In the case of patients admitted into intensive care units, with death as the most likely outcome, in order to avoid 'suffering' by the patient, prolonged emotional trauma to the close relatives and waste of resources, more and more doctors tend to decide not to resuscitate, if cardiopulmonary function stops.

LIVING WILL

Some persons prepare living wills in advance of the onset of serious illness. The living will gives the preference of the person at the time of making it of future action under certain foreseen or unforeseen circumstances. The California National Act (1977) recognised the living will: "If at any time, I should suffer from an incurable disease or injury and it should be medically determined that any treatment would only prolong my dying, I direct that life sustaining treatment be withheld or withdrawn and that I may be permitted to die a natural death aided only by those measures that are necessary for my comfort".

The living will (advance directives) for health care is a statement, usually in writing, in which the patient extends his/

her right to refuse any proposed treatment (autonomy) to a future time, when he/she may not be fully mentally competent.

An advance directive is usually given when an acute clinical episode occurs in a patient with a long-standing or progressive condition, which has already compromised the quality of life. The background condition may be dementia, or terminal and progressive degenerative diseases, such as malignancy or neuromuscular disorders. Decisions to withhold active treatment should always be made with the understanding that nursing care and symptomatic therapy will always be continued.

People who make an advance directive should inform chosen relatives or friends (and their family doctor and legal advisor, if they have any). Ideally, people who have written an advance directive should carry a card indicating that fact.

The living will is not legal here and not binding on the doctors. The preference of the patient might have changed with the changes in circumstances. It is not an uncommon experience to see that the patient who had previously stated that particular procedures be not done on him, being thankful for the same procedure for saving his life. The doctor must act in the best interest of the patient, taking into consideration the present condition, the patient's wishes and possibilities of recovery of function and health.

A 70-year-old male, a hypertensive, who had a mild stroke earlier, has another stroke, leading to extensive paralysis and loss of speech and memory. The patient is unable to communicate now. His son brings a "living will" dated 6 months earlier (after the mild stroke). It says that no active treatment be given if he suffers from another stroke".

What should the doctor do? Should he accept the living will and refrain from active treatment? The doctor should reassess the situation and make a decision, taking into consideration all factors. The patient's wish as expressed in the 'will' is only one of the many factors helping to make a decision.

What is the ancient teaching with respect to the terminally ill?

Tatvat pratikriya karya yavac chavasiti manavah

(As long as the patient breathes, so long provide treatment)

There is the opposing instruction:

Upekshanam prakristhesu

(Withdraw treatment in the moribund patient)

The two apparently contradictory advices probably mean that specific treatment against the particular disease is to be given up but treatment (care) aimed at reducing suffering and giving comfort should be continued. Efforts must be made always to achieve peaceful death with comfort once it is decided that the person is having an irreversible terminal illness.

QUALITY OF LIFE

The purpose of medicine is to improve the quality of life. Where there is threat to life, it attempts to prevent death; where there is pain or other undesirable symptoms, it brings about relief of the symptoms; where there is compromised functions, it tries to support these functions and prevent or delay further deterioration. Medicine thus tries to enhance the quality of life.

The term "Quality of Life" is difficult to define. It is subjective. It depends on the perception of the person who evaluates "quality". It could be the patient, the health professional, a relative or an onlooker.

Quality of life may refer to:

1. subjective satisfaction experienced by the person (such satisfaction has physical, mental, social and spiritual dimensions), or
2. objective achievement of attributes and skills.

We say that the quality of life is poor when it falls below a certain standard (never absolute) in a particular person. It can be loss of mobility, vision or hearing. It could be pain. It could be deterioration of mental ability. It may be inability to interact socially or spiritually.

There was an air-force pilot who had to bail out and sustained fracture of spine leading to paraplegia. People remarked "What a terrible thing to happen; what a future". But the former pilot readjusted himself. He was more active, becoming the secretary of the Red Cross Society, though confined to the wheelchair.

There was a young doctor, who had an accident, leading to paraplegia. She did not give up. Her biography is given in the book "Take my Hands". By her continued and devoted work, deriving immense pleasure, she has shown how the quality of life was satisfying.

To the onlooker,the quality of life was poor in both instances. But to the concerned persons, the quality of life was good and eminently satisfying in the service of the people.

The attending doctor must not jump to conclusions regarding quality of life. The doctor's duty is to assess the situation and improve the quality to the maximum extent possible.

Sometimes the discussions on the quality of life come up when an ethical decision has to be taken whether to continue life-suport or not. In most of such cases, the patient may not be in a position to express his views and preferences. Often, the question is asked: Is such a life worth living? Is quality of life as seen by the treating doctor or others, the decisive factor in making a decision to withhold or withdraw interventions necessary for life? Is there a minimum threshold of quality of life below which life is not worth sustaining?

PERSISTENT VEGETATIVE STATE

People may lose their cerebral cortical functions and remain in a vegetative state. Most of them are caused by:
- head injury
- hypoxia of the cerebral cortex due to cardiac arrest or hypotension, or
- hypoglycemic crises in diabetic patients.

In such patients,
- the eyes may be open and may turn to light or sound, but there is no cognition,
- the patient may respond reflexly to painful stimuli, by withdrawing the limb or grimacing of face, but the patient may not be suffering from pain,
- there is no voluntary activity, and
- there is no meaningful response to environment.

The chances of the person regaining consciousness after 3 months of such a state are minimal. In the few instances recorded of regaining consciousness, the person was severely physically handicapped, mentally disabled and dependent on others for all functions. A person in the vegetative state may, however, live for years. They are neither suffering (apparently) nor are they terminally ill.

What is to be done in such instances? The family may request that the agony of watching the person in the vegetative state be ended and that all support to the patient be withdrawn.

There were no specific guidelines in India till the supreme court judgement in Aruna Shanbaug case.

Aruna Shanbaug was sexually assaulted by a safai karamchari at the KEM Hospital. He choked her with a dog chain and raped her. She was brain dead due to asphyxiation. She was in a vegetative state since then.

The Supreme Court legalized passive euthanasia by means of withdrawal of life support to patients in a permanent vegetative state. However certain guidelines were laid down viz

a. Decision to discontinue life support can be taken by: (i) parents, (ii) spouse, (iii) close relative, (iv) friend, in case none of earlier 3 available, and (v) doctors attending the patient.
b. Decision should be taken bonafide in the best interest of the patient.
c. Decision requires approval from High Court.
d. Chief justice of High Court constitute a bench of at least two judges.
e. A committe of three reputed doctors to be nominated by bench.
f. Before giving verdict a notice regarding the report should be given to close relatives and the state.
g. After hearing the parties, the High Court can give its verdict.

Hospice

When patients are beyond active medical treatment, there is still a place for caring—the hospice. The most valuable treatment here is *tender loving care*. Relief of pain and other symptomatic treatment are also given. One such hospice is the "Shanti Avedna Ashram" in Mumbai, where a caring team of sisters and volunteers provide compassionate care to the terminally ill.

CHAPTER 13

Euthanasia

Euthanasia means "good death". The term "euthanasia" is derived from two Greek words: *'eu'* = good and *'thanatos'* = death. It means "voluntary putting to death of a patient who is suffering from an incurable, terminal and extremely painful condition". It has been called "mercy killing", i.e. "death without suffering".

CLASSIFICATION

According to the Will of the Patient

Voluntary Euthanasia

The patient (the sufferer) requests for the termination of his/her life and gives free consent for it. It is often referred to as 'assisted suicide'. Some people call it 'homicide by request'. It is legal in countries like Belgium, Luxembourg, Netherlands, Switzerland, US (Oregon and Washington).

Non-voluntary Euthanasia

The decision to end the life of the sufferer is not taken by the individual but by the society or a group of individuals, or a person close to the sufferer. The sufferer is not in a position to signify his/her volition. The wish of the patient may not be known; the patient may be in irreversible coma.

Involuntary Euthanasia

Patient does not want to die, yet he is compulsorily killed.

According to Physician's Act

Active Euthanasia

In active euthanasia, on the request of the patient that his/her life be ended, the doctor, or nurse, or a similar person administers a lethal agent, with the intention of causing death. The advocates of euthanasia argue that the right to die is implicit in the right of life. They ask that the mentally competent person be given the freedom to make a choice whether to live or to die.

As the law stands today, no one has the right to do away with-life, whether one' sown or that of any other, except under certain conditions such as war or after due process of law as a punishment. *Life isinviolable.*

Medical teaching has always emphasized the need for preservation of life. Hippocratic oath says:"Neither will I administer a poison to anybody when asked to do so, nor will I suggest such a course".

Deliberately causing the death of another person constitutes a criminal act (homicide), as does cooperating in causing another's death. All ethical codes reject euthanasia. The law forbids it.

Ramanujam, a 53 years old male, with cancer lung and bony metastases, has no hope of recovery. He does not want to continue to suffer. He requests the doctor to put an end to his life.

Patients make requests for swift death to escape from pain and suffering. The patients also do not want to be a burden on their family. They do not want to be dependent on others. There is an increasing demand for "death with dignity". The patient (and often the relatives) desires to be spared the pain and inconveniences of repeated interventions which bring little comfort. "Death with dignity" emphasies the need to care for the patient in increasing manner.We have today the means to control pain and suffering. The hospice movement has been very beneficial.

Active euthanasia variants

In West Germany, a doctor attending a patient desirous of puttingan end to life, made available a potent life-taking drink, to be taken by the patient if the patient so desired. The drink was left on the side table. Both the doctor and the patient knew the purpose. After the doctor left the room, the patient drank the mixture, ending her life.

In this case, the doctor was accessory to bringing about the death actively. The motive was clear. In the United States of America, Dr Jack Kevorkian developed what he calls, the "death machine", causing the death of many persons. Heeven gave a demonstration on television. He was then prosecuted and punished with long jailsentence.

Passive Euthanasia

In passive euthanasia, there is no active intervention to end life. The doctor stands by "passively", allowing nature to take its course. No specific medication is given against the progress of the disease. Life supporting measures are also avoided.

Patient Ramanujam comes to a stage, where his respiratory function has deteriorated to such an extent that he can survive only by artificial life support systems and resuscitative measures. Considering all aspects and after consultations with all people concerned, a decision is taken not to resuscitate. The decision is documented. No resuscitation measures are used. The patient dies.

In the case of Ramanujam, the procedure of active resuscitation was omitted and the patient died. If, on the other hand, it had been decided to resuscitate him and later, the respirator was turned off, it will be an act of commission. Broadly active euthanasia is killing while passive euthanasia is letting die.

Passive euthanasia is legal in India since 7 march 2011 after supreme court judgment in **Aruna Shanbaug case**. *Citation- Aruna Ramchandra Shanbaug vs Union of India, (2011) 4 SCC 454.*

There are a number of considerations:

1. Autonomy of the patient: Freedom to make choices in accordance with his/her own values. A competent patient has the right to for ego life-sustainingtreatment.
2. Beneficence: Failure to save a patient's life (when that is possible) is contrary to the principle of beneficence.
3. Non-maleficence: A treatment that is likely to end in the death of the patient generally violates the principle of non-maleficence.
4. Potential consequences of the policy being adopted and societal consequences.

When the patient is in the terminal stage, there is no need for heroic treatment but ordinary treatment should be continued. This will be based on customariness, naturalness, complexity, expense of treatment, invasiveness, burdens of the treatment and balance of likely benefits.

All consensus today is that unnecessary prolongation of life (death) is to be avoided. Decisions must be taken in advance in each individual case.

The following procedures can be avoided:

1. Emergency resuscitation after cardiac arrest in the terminally ill,
2. Treatment of serious pulmonary infections in patients with painful terminal illness, and
3. Continuation of artificial life support for patients with extensive brain damage.

All patients who are not terminally ill and who experience unexpected cardiopulmonary arrest or difficulty must be resuscitated. Other considerations such as age and mental illness or mental retardation do not come into reckoning to withhold cardiopulmonary resuscitation. So also, chronic illness, which can be treated, should not be a ground for denying cardiopulmonary resuscitation.

In the termination of life, there can be conflict of interest:

- The family of the patient may want to terminate the agonising watch.
- Those interested in organ transplantation may press for a new approach to"death".
- Society may have a vested interest in terminating a costly procedure in what is considered a "hopeless case".
- There may be competing cases for the use of the same respirator or other service resources.
- There can be selfish rationalization by the patients, relatives or the hospital authorities.
- The patients might be influenced by the worry about the trouble they are causing their family, and a sense of guilt at being a live.

Dr HS, a practitioner in Manchester, UK, treating mainly elderly women, was accused of killing more than 115 women by injecting diamorphine, between March 1995 and June 1998. Police tracked more than 100 dead bodies with prima facie evidence that the doctor was involved in all these killings. He was sentenced to life imprisonment; his name was erased from the register of the General Medical Council.

A cautious approach is needed. Euthanasia can be misused. The euthanasia program initiated in Germany in the early 1930's had the support of many well-meaning doctors. It was first directed at the incurably ill. Later it gradually expanded and deteriorated into genocide.

The psychiatrists who supervised the killings in the cyanide gas filled cells at Hadamar Mental Institute in Germany were condemned to death in the Neuremberg trials (1945). The British Medical Association then declared: "They (the doctors) departed from the traditional medical ethics which maintains the value and sanctity of every individual human being they betrayed the trust society had placed in them as a profession".

The British Medical Association set up a Working Party to reconsider its policy on euthanasia. They concluded (1988): "The law should not be changed and the deliberate taking of a human life should remain.a crime. This rejection of a change in the law is.... affirmation of the supreme value of the individual, no matter how worthless others and that individual mayfeel".

The World Medical Association (1987) declared: "Euthanasia, that is the act of deliberately ending the life of a patient, either at his own request or at the request of close relatives, is unethical".

Recentlya US Federal Appeals Courtruled that the mentally competent, terminally ill patients have the right to a doctor's assistance in hastening their deaths. A patient has "a strong liberty interest in choosing a dignified and humane death rather than being reduced at the end of his existence to a child-like state of helplessness, diapered, sedated and incompetent". The American Medical Association opposed the decision and issued an official statement: "We would stand by our stance that it would be unethical for a physician to participate in an assisted suicide, which would be the active killing of a patient" — as reported in the British Medical Journal, 12: 216,1996.

In Netherlands, the law did not (till recently) permit euthanasia but no legal action was taken, if specific conditions were followed. In 1997, 6000 out of about 9000 requests for euthanasia were turned down, because:

- suffering was not unbearable;
- it could be palliated;
- available treatment had not been completed; or
- there was evidence of treatable depression.

The Netherlands Parliament has now made euthanasia legal under specified conditions.

"Dutch Senate passes Euthanasia bill"
—The Hindu, Bombay, 12 April 2001.

"The Upper House (Senate) in Holland took a historic decision today when with a vote of 46 to 28, it passed the euthanasia bill".

"In December, the Dutch Lower House had approved the euthanasia bill by 104 votes to 40. Under the new law, patients over the age of 16 who suffer from acute and unremitting pain can ask doctors to end their lives, although under strict medical and legal guidelines".

MEDICINE, LAW AND THEOLOGY

The three disciplines concerned with the problem of euthanasia are Medicine, Law and Theology. The person involved has three relationships: to his/her own self; to his/her doctor; and to the society. The doctor has similarly responsibilities to the sick person and to the society. The society is interested in the 'individual good' of the patient and the 'common good' of the society.

Medical teaching has always emphasized the need for preservation of life. It has, down the ages, rejected the direct taking of life. To ask the doctor, who guards life, to be the executor of life, would affect the ethos of the profession. It can destroy the relationship of trust that should characterize the relationship between the patient and the doctor. The doctor takes the Hippocratic Oath (often a modified version) at the time of graduation/registration with the Medical Council. That Oath commits the doctor against the taking of life. The International Code of Medical Ethics (1983) says: "Aphysician shall always bear in mind the obligation of preserving human life."

Euthanasia is condemned by most religions; they favor natural death. We do not have the authority to take innocent life (exceptions: death by law, death in military action). Any killing of the innocent is wrong and against 'natural law'. Further, many religions believe that human suffering has certain values; it helps him/her to be spiritually uplifted.

Does the right to life include a right to die? In Smt Gian Kaur-*vs*-State of Punjab, the Supreme Court (1996 Cri. L.J. 1960) has laid down the law that by no stretch of imagination could the 'extinction of life' be read into the 'right to life' contained in Article 21 of the constitution. The right to life is a *natural right* whereas the taking away of life is an *unnatural* termination of life and hence inconsistent and incompatible with the right to life. Does this conflict with 'autonomy', one of the cardinal principles of medical ethics? This is where the hierarchy of ethical principles comes: the preservation of life takes precedence.

THE AGED

"Aged Americans to the bin", so runs the headlines of an article quoted in Sunday Herald of September 22, 1991. The article reads:

"Elderly and frail Americans are being abandoned at hospital emergency rooms in a new phenomenon known as "granny dumping", according to the American Association for Retired Persons".

When values are eroded, the first to be affected are those at either end of the spectrum of life.

SUICIDE

Suicide is often an act of despair. The person has failed to find meaning in his or her life or has muddled it and made continuation of life senseless (to him or her). There may be acute mental disturbances (most often depression) in some persons. Sometimes persons tend to resort to suicide because they feel rejected by their family or society. The blame could well be with the society. It is necessary to help the person attempting suicide to find sense in his or her life.

Suicide in India is criminal. Attempt at suicide is punishable. There are people who question this attitude. The Indian Law Commission, in its 42nd report, has stated: "It is a monstrous procedure to inflict further suffering in the individual who has already found life so miserable, his chances of happiness as slender, that he has been willing to face pain and death to cease living".

Attempt at suicide is often a call for help. That call must be responded.

The medical profession must try to identify the concerns the person's requests for assisted suicide. Appropriate response by good support, comfort, good communication and adequate pain-control will reduce the request for euthanasia and assisted suicide.

Section 6: Health Policy and Health Care

CHAPTER 14 Health Policy

Most decisions on health policy raise ethical questions. The health policy of a state or a nation depends on its value systems. The health policy defines the strategies for optimising the social uses of the body of knowledge in the field of medicine and health and of the resources available.

A look at the health policy can give us an idea of the values upheld by the country and the people. Does that policy provide care for the disadvantaged and the vulnerable? Does it give priority to the care of the very young, the aged , the poor, the marginalized and the disabled? Does that policy provide care only or mostly for those who can buy that care? What is the mix?

The Government of India statement on National Health Policy (1982) starts with "The constitution of India envisages the establishment of a new social order based on equality, freedom, justice and the dignity of the individual. It aims at the elimination of poverty, ignorance and ill-health and directs the State to regard the raising of the level of nutrition and the standard of living of its people and the improvement of public health among its primary duties, securing the health and strength of the workers, men and women, specially ensuring the children are given opportunities and facilities to development in a healthy manner". The statement goes on to analyse the present situation and states that the health picture of the country still "constitutes a cause for serious and urgent concern". It further states: "Presently, despite the constraint of resources, there is disproportionate emphasis on the establishment of curative centers—dispensaries, hospitals, institutions for specialist treatment—the large majority of which are located in the urban areas of the country".

We are conscious of our poverty and lack of resources. Yet, often we find large sums of money invested in sophisticated technologies. These are expensive. The Government of India Health Policy states: "The existing situation has been largely engendered by the almost wholesale adoption of health manpower development policies and the establishment of curative centers based on the Western models, which are inappropriate and irrelevant to the real needs of our people and the socioeconomic conditions obtaining in the country. The hospital-based, disease and cure-oriented approach towards the establishment of medical sevices has provided benefits to the upper crusts of society, specially those residing in urban areas".

Other countries are also considering these issues. The conference on philosphy of Medicine held in Canton, China (1979) consisered two issues in medical ethics:

- Concept of death and euthanasia, and
- Delivery of medical care without discrimination.

In the USA also, there is rethinking.

CHOICES

When the resources are limited, choices have to be made. Can there be rationing of medical care? Should not the care go to the most needy? Should the resources be allocated such that the maximum benefit goes to the maximum number of people? At the same time, the doctor is committed to give the best possible care to the patient under his/her care. The doctor does not want any curtailment of the freedom of the doctor and the patient to choose the best care for the individual. These choices are hard to make. How they are made depends on the dominant value systems. One or other group will consider itself in a disadvantaged position.

The tensions between 'individual good' and 'social good' occur in every society and affect the decisions. There will be demands for:

1. more and better medical care and services for the individual, and
2. more fair distribution of the benefits of medical and health care among all.

The traditional viewpoint is that the doctor is mostly concemed with the patient under his/her care. He/she is accountable to the individual patient, providing the best possible care, irrepective of other consideration. The policy maker is accountable to the public and the society. Should the doctor be involved in policy-making or only in the implemention of the policy made by others? Very often, the view is taken that it is for the health administrators (ministers, secretaries to government, planning committees and others in the case of central/state governments and the management and chief executives in the case of institutions/organisations) to make the policy; once the policy is made, the clinician should have the freedom to act as he/she thinks best within that policy.

Society is a collection of individuals. If we could give maximum care for every individual in the society, it would have been ideal. But we cannot. We do not have the resources. We tend to pour the available resources into the care of some individuals even though expectations of benefit are low. Other individuals with great possibilities of benefit, get little share of the resources. There is always conflict between different groups as regards health care—rich versus poor; old versus young; aggressive versus passive patients. When one group receives a disproportionate amount of resources compared to another group, society suffers.

In making the health policy, many factors come into play:

- medical and healthcare indications,
- availability of medical and health interventions for the individual and the society,
- patient and doctor preferences,
- improvement of the quality of life of the individual and the society,
- values held by the society, such as justice,
- cost to the individual and to the society, and
- overall good of the society.

In India, the resources are very limited. A choice has to be made between the demands of the few to get the 'best' possible care for the individual and the needs of many to get at least the 'basic' care. There are diseases of affluence and diseases of poverty.

Health policy has to address many questions:

- Who shall receive what health care?
- What resources can be allocated to health in comparison to other sectors?
- How shall the resources be allocated within the health sector?
- How do we set our priorities?
- Who shall decide on health policy? How are the policy makers to be chosen? What role shall the doctors have in the making of the policy?

- Should there be control of the use of expensive medical technology in the management of the individual patient?
- Should there be a cost containment programme?

The Washington Post, April 27, 1990

"In a major break from the long dominant position of organized medicine, the American College of Physicians, the nation's largest group of specialists, called yesterday for a radical restructuring of costly and uneven American healthcare system to guarantee equal access for all Americans". The statement said that "The current situation is intolerable for patients, their families and physicians". The American College of Physicians sought to determine a single standard of quality care that should be available to all Americans, regardless of their financial status. An important feature was the statement that the medical profession "bears responsibility" to ensure that "acceptable, appropriate and cost-effective care is to be delivered".

The above statement reflects a departure from the oft-repeated thinking that the maximum good of the individual is the goal of medical care. It places the responsibility on the doctor to ensure that health care be made available to all of a uniform standard of quality and which is acceptable, appropriate and cost-effective.

There is need to reflect on the value of human life and its intrinsic worth. Is a 25-year-old man, earning the livelihood for his family more valuable than a 70-year-old pensioner? If they are both admitted to the hospital and both require the ventilator and only one is available, who should get it? If the 70-year-old man is a poet, will it alter the situation? If the person is a minister in the Government, would it alter the priorities in medical care? Would priorities be based on fame, wealth, influence, or responsibility for many?

There is need for the doctors in India to address these and many similar issues. What is the health care which must be available to all, regardless of the situation, ability to pay and other factors? The society must assure this level of care. The health policy of the country must reflect it.

THE SCOPE

The health policy should ensure a minimum (basic) acceptable level of care. What should it include?

1. Caring.
2. Promotion of health by improving lifestyles. Health education plays an important role.
3. Prevention of diseases—better water supply and sanitation, immunization, campaigns, such as those against smoking, alcohol and drug abuse, accident prevention, and legislation.
4. Primary health care and emergency care.
5. Reducing the burden of infections and other preventable diseases and premature death.
6. Individualized forms of care to deal with common illnesses and compatible with a reasonable allocation of resources to health sector.

In determining the individualized forms of care, a question arises. Is a particular medical intervention "basic"? The answer depends on:

- benefits and risks;
- health outcome;
- cost (cost:benefit ratio, cost-effectiveness ratio); and
- number of persons benefitting.

Interventions which have great benefits, very little risks, good health outcomes, low costs and benefitting many people will be included in the basic care to be provided. Interventions which have low levels of benefits, high levels of risks, are costly and benefit only a few cannot be considered as basic. It may be essential from a particular patient's point of view but it is not basic with respect to the health policy. It is often difficult to decide whether a particular intervention is basic or not but the decision has to be made.

Who shall decide whether a particular intervention is basic or essential? Many groups or representatives must be involved in the decision-making and laying down of the policy. First will be the persons who are likely to receive the benefit. These are the public-patients or would be patients. Among them will be the affluent and the poor. They will have different perceptions. To the affluent a costly intervention may still appear 'basic'. To the poor, even an apparently not-so-costly intervention may appear as costly and, therefore, not 'basic'. How to get a representative group? Probably people with a median financial status or income or net worth could be included. Other factors which should be considered in the selection of representatives include education, occupation, belief, values and geography. Another question is : how many? Too few will not be representative enough; too many will make it unwieldy.

Another representation will be those who provide the care. These would include the medical, nursing and other health professionals and those belonging to the allied professions. They could provide the cost-benefit and cost-effectiveness of the interventions and the health outcomes.

Those who meet the cost should be represented. These include the Government (Central, State and others) and managements of voluntary agencies. The patients (already included in the first group) are also people who meet the costs, when there is payment for service.

Once we have decided on the basic (minimum) level of health care, other questions arise:

If the minimum care is provided for all, can some people receive (buy) a higher level of care, because they are rich/influential/ powerful or have a higher social worth?

The Charter of Health Promotion of the World Health Organization (Ottawa, 1986) has a pledge to:

- move into the arena of healthy public policy, and to advocate a clear political commitment to health and equity in all sectors;
- counteract the pressures towards harmful products, resource depletion, unhealthy living conditions and environments and bad nutrition and to focus attention on public health issues, such as pollution, occupational hazards, housing and settlements;
- respond to health gap within and between societies and tackle the inequities in health, living conditions and well-being;
- reorient health services and their resources towards the promotion of health and share power with other sectors, other disciplines and most importantly with people themselves;
- recognize health and its maintenance as a major social investment and challenge and address the overall ecological issue of our ways of living.

A purely medical response will not bring about a solution to the problems in health care. There has to be interaction between medicine and politics. Political unrest, terrorism, natural disasters, poverty, economic incompetence and misuse of funds create crises in health in addition to the usual causes of diseases—infectious, degenerative, nutritional and others. It is useless knowing that many diseases are preventable unless we act on that knowledge.

Knowing that proper antenatal care will reduce infant mortality is of no use, if we do not take the necessary action. Health professionals have to participate in political decisions. We have to help shape the decisions to bring about better health.

THE COMMON GOOD

A concept which is important in determining the policy is the "The Common Good". The aim is to bring as much all round benefit as possible to the majority; at the same time, it should not cause undue suffering to the minority. It tries to ensure maximum amount of happiness for the greatest number of people. Every person must receive the care that the person needs. The principle of equitable distribution of medical and health care according to need must be followed. It requires a comprehensive health service designed to meet the needs of all the people within the existing constraints.

The medical profession in our country must address itself to the priorities in medical care. Decisions must be taken as to how the resources available are to be utilized. Should it be on getting sophisticated equipment and developing centers to manage degenerative diseases (for such procedures as coronary bypass surgery) or should priority be given to treat the common communicable diseases, rampant in the country? The debate will go on. Shall the State establish three more centres for kidney transplantation or utilise that money and resources in the management of 30,000 children with diarrhoea? Shall the State build speciality and subspeciality/superspeciality centers, with the costly, sophisticated, imported technology to take care of the few, when the Government hospitals are overcrowded with two patients in one bed or patients lying on the floor in the corridors and in urgent need for care for the common but serious ailments? The doctors will have to make the choice and advise the Government on the choices.

Public Health

All public health policies should follow the cardinal principles of medical ethics.

- *Beneficence* : The policy, when implemented, should benefit all the people, or at least, the large majority of the people and not merely select groups at the expense of the rest.

- *Non-maleficence*: The programs/projects should not harm anyone. When framing the policy, the possibility of causing harm in the short- or long-term must be considered carefully.
- *Justice*: There should not be any discrimination; there should be no injustice done to anyone.
- *Autonomy*: There should be no violation of the rights.

The Medical profession has a responsibility to improve the health of the population. The profession must actively participate in the production of an appropriate policy on public health and its implementation, monitoring and evaluation. Producing a policy paper on public health without ensuring its implementation is unethical; it raises false hopes.

CHAPTER 15

Distributive Justice in Health Care

RIGHT TO HEALTH

Is there a right to health? Article. 35 of the Universal declaration of human rights states:

"Everyone has the right to a standard of living adequate for the health and well-being of himself and his family including food, clothing, housing and medical care and necessary social services". The Alma Ata conference declared: "Governments have a responsibility for the health of the people, which can be fulfilled only by adequate and equitably distributed health and social measures". Health does not figure as a fundamental right in the Indian Constitution. But it is present in the Directive Principles of State Policy (considered as the conscience of the Constitution). Article 39 of the Constitution requires the State to make policies to ensure health. Article 47 makes it obligatory for the State to make improvements in public health.

If there is a right to health (and it appears to be so from the various statements), it is the duty of the State (and the people) to ensure that a standard of health care adequate to maintain the health of the people is provided. The healthcare services should not fall below it.

The present situation is deplorable. Large sections of the people live in conditions where it is not possible to have healthy living. There is no proper supply of water. Sanitation does not exist. There is no housing. It is no wonder that they die young (infant and child mortality). Nutrition is poor. Instead of growing food which the people of the place can eat, crops are grown to earn some money.

It is not enough to take measures to provide health care. It is necessary to assure quality of the care being provided.

Many countries are taking action to ensure quality care of the health of the people. The WHO regional office for Europe decided in 1984:

> "By 1990 all member States should have built effective mechanisms for ensuring quality of patient care within their health care systems. This could be achieved by establishing methods and procedures for systematically monitoring the quality of care given to patients and making assessment and regulation a permanent component of health professionals' regular activities, providing all health personnel with training in quality assurance".

What is the present position in India? There is negation of the right to health. With a little effort on the part of the Government, it is possible to bring about large scale improvements in health. Vitamin A deficiency causes blindness; the children become more prone to and succumb from infection. Do they not have the right to be provided adequate intake of vitamin by better nutrition or by supplements? What is the role of the doctor in preventing or making good such deficiencies? There are nearly 300 million people living in iodine deficient areas. Should they not be protected against the deficiency? The doctors know of the deficiencies. Is it ethical to remain quiet, when correction is simple and within the resources of the State?

DISTRIBUTIVE JUSTICE

Health care in an unjust society cannot be just. Yet health is an area which can lead to a more just society.

Even in countries where the total resources are good and the allocation of funds to the health sector is relatively high, the distribution of healthcare services is often unsatisfactory. There is disparity between groups of people and between regions. A better distribution is necessary. When we come to poor countries like India, where the resources are far from being satisfactory and allocation to the health sector is meagre, it is essential to provide as fair a distribution as possible. The greatest medical ethical need in India today is probably justice and equity in the allocation of resources and distribution of healthcare services. There is need for the use of the limited available resources for the benefit of all. The capacity of the majority of people to "purchase" healthcare services is limited. The availability is also restricted. Ethically, it is necessary to provide a just distribution of healthcare services ensuring accessibility and affordability. Whatever be the resources or means available, they must be distributed without discrimination.

The health situation in the country shows wide and intolerable disparities. Any indicator can be taken and the wide variation becomes evident immediately.

Infant mortality rate (1988):
Kerala : 29
All India : 96
Uttar Pradesh : 126

There are disparities between the urban and the rural and between male and female.

Infant mortality rate (1988):
Rural : 105
Urban : 62

There are again marked differences if we consider the tribal areas. The health of the people in the tribal areas is much worse. There is also need to give special consideration to high-risk and vulnerable groups, such as children, mothers, pregnant women and the elderly.

But the most important factor producing differences in health is the economic condition. There is disproportionate investment of personnel and other resources catering to the affluent. The rich and the powerful often get far better health care than the poor and marginalized. Should medical care take into consideration the social worth or contribution (past, present or future) of the person to the society? Can there be reverse discrimination in favor of the poor, the weak and the neglected?

> "The people in a civilized state may be divided into many different orders but for the purpose of investigating the manner in which they enjoy or are deprived of the requisite to support the health of their bodies and minds, they need only be divided into two classes, viz. the rich and the poor".
>
> —Charles Hill (1805)

This is true of India today. The health gap between the rich and the poor, the skilled and the unskilled, the employed (especially in the organized sector) and the unemployed is very wide. Poverty and unemployment with poor nutrition, poor provision of medical care, dilapidated housing or no housing, and substandard or no education all contribute to poor health. Poverty is the greatest threat to health and this is especially so with respect to the health of women and infants who are the first to suffer.

Substantial health benefits could be expected to accrue from a policy of better income distribution.

There is need for equity in health. We can reduce the gap between the 'haves' and the 'have nots' in different ways:

- Reduce deprivation. Ensure the minimum requirements.
- Reduce health inequality.

There is need for direct investment in the health of all the people. One way of ensuring better distribution is to make greater efforts on promotive and preventive care. They can be expected to yield better dividends, irrespective of the person's capacity to pay. These can be in the areas of water supply, sanitation and waste disposal, prevention of environmental pollution and the expanded program of immunization. In addition, there ought to be greater emphasis and better allocation of resources to primary health care. Establishing more primary health centers and subcenters in rural and tribal areas and ensuring that they are fully staffed and equipped with necessary infrastructure would help to reduce the urban bias, so evident today.

There are many areas which are underserved with respect to health personnel. Can it be made mandatory for a doctor to serve in such areas for a minimum period of time? Is it ethical to force a doctor to serve in underserved areas against his/her will? Is it ethical for a doctor to refuse to serve in such an area, in view of the advantages he/she had received? Is it not to be expected that the doctor will give his or her services to the needy in return for the privileges received by way of education and facilities including the "use" of patients to gain skills and experience?

CHAPTER 16

Technology

The modern world is shaped to a large extent by technology. The world shaped by technology is becoming more and more inhuman. Can we have a *technology* with a human face, as EG Schumacher says in *Small is beautiful*? Nature knows when and where to stop. Not so technology. It does not recognize the self-limiting principle. Technology, though a product of man, tends to develop its own laws and principles, different from those of human nature. It leads to a way of life based on materialism. Inappropriate use of technology in the medical field, tends to remove the personal humane approach to people needing health care.

There is worldwide a sudden surge of sophisticated, costly medical technology, both diagnostic and therapeutic. The costly equipments are marketed aggressively. There are acute pressures from different interest groups: The manufacturers and their representatives; the doctor who wants to have the latest technologies and equipment; the public who are made aware of the newer additions by the mass media. The high pressure advertisements make the profession and the public feel that there is need for getting all these investigations done. The market in medical equipment is currently estimated at between Rupees two hundred and fifty crores and three hundred crores, with an annual growth rate of 20-25%.

High technology medical care has come into India with a bang in recent times. This is welcomed in certain circles, especially the highly affluent and in the industries and financial institutions because of the high profits. It is producing disquiet and anxiety in the majority of the people. It increases the gap between the 'haves' and the 'have nots'.

DIAGNOSTIC TECHNOLOGY

The development of modern diagnostic techniques is phenomenal. They often *supplant*, rather than *supplement*, the clinical examination. It is often forgotten that the careful clinical examination remains the cornerstone of diagnosis and assessment. A carefully taken history and properly conducted physical examination yield good results and are often sufficient. But there is an increasing tendency to carry out expensive, uncomfortable and occasionally even hazardous procedures unnecessarily to establish or confirm the diagnosis. Sometimes, these newer diagnostic techniques only confuse the issues and lead to wrong decision.

There is continuous search for ultimate accuracy in diagnosis. The newer alternatives being offered are most often extremely costly and beyond the reach of the individual, family, community and Government. They consume large proportion of resources. It is necessary that we control this costly process, when there are more crying needs. Cost-benefit and cost-effectiveness analyses call for a stop to this onrush for costlier diagnostic technology with limited use. It is an ethical problem.

An endless array of newer diagnostic modalities come up all the time. Highly sophisticated, capital intensive equipments like magnetic resonance imaging, positron emission tomography, cardiac catheterization laboratory, and laser technology are used. There is also rapid development in technology with early obsolescence. The cost is high.

Many of the doctors qualified abroad and returning to India are often dependent on the highly sophisticated equipment to which they were accustomed when they were abroad. They demand such equipment and tests. Some of them maintain links with the institutions where they had worked and continue to feel that equipment available there should be available in India also, forgetting the socioeconomic and technological differences. We are not able to provide even the ordinary tests for all the people. We are not able to maintain the sophisticated equipment, imported at great cost.

While all diagnostic technologies suffer from the problems of escalating costs, it is most acute in the case of the imaging technologies. Most of the people in India cannot have the benefit of even the simplest X-ray examination. But now, there is demand for ultrasound, CT scanning and magnetic resonance imaging. CT scanning and magnetic resonance imaging represent quantum jumps in expenses over the routine radiology and ultrasound. Among the other non-invasive techniques of diagnostic procedures are echocardiography, computerized stress testing, color doppler, nuclear medicine and mammography. Invasive ones include cardiac catheterization and coronary and other angiographies.

Dilemma: To do the best for the individual patient irrespective of cost *versus* the duty to do the best for all patients within the constraints of the resources.

Even in the most affluent countries, the financial facts put limits to the use of the newer, costlier technologies.

Cascade Effect of Tests

Many of the tests, using the sophisticated technologies, do not yield conclusive results. One test leads on to another. Right or wrong, the test result introduces a doubt that must be resolved by further testing. The danger is that the cascade effect may be triggered by an inappropriate test in the first instance. It then becomes difficult to stop. We place too much reliance on technology. A common experience is with the use of electronic fetal monitoring in obstetrics. Electronic fetal monitoring has replaced or is threatening to replace personal attention at the bedside of the woman in labor. It has contributed to the staggering increase in cesarian sections. According to various evaluations, the device does not offer any advantage to mother or child.

The limitations of the laboratory tests are not understood or considered seriously. There can be many false negatives and false positives.

The blood of the would be donor (relative of the patient) was sent for HIV test; the ELISA test came as positive. Even before the confirmatory test was done, the result became known. It created a lot of personal, family and social problems. The donor, however, would not accept the result. The ELISA test was repeated in three different laboratories. All of them came as negative.

Normal findings may be obtained in ill-heafth; findings beyond the average range may be seen in a healthy person. Sophisticated equipment need skilled maintenance. Quality control and calibration are a must for any equipment or procedure, but are not done many a time. Simple changes in the voltage of the current can lead to bizarre results.

The person who interprets the results has limitations. Variations are very common in the interpretation of the findings by different radiologists, ultrasonologists and others.

CURATIVE TECHNOLOGY

The curative technologies have also shown changes. These are mainly in the development of newer drugs, sophisticated life support systems and surgical techniques, such as open heart surgery and organ transplantation. Such technology might benefit a few for sometime but the cost is so high that such procedures are out of the reach of most people.

There are many newer drugs like antibiotics or antihypertensives coming up all the time. One common finding is that the cost of management increases. When a newer antibiotic comes into the market, it is used indiscriminately and in preference to others (because it has a broader spectrum of sensitivity). The organisms soon develop resistance. Still newer antibiotics are needed. One sad example is enteric fever. Because of the indiscriminate use of chloramphenicol for all sorts of infections, we are unable to manage enteric fever with it. Newer, more powerful and more costly antibiotics are needed. Even they do not produce the desired results. Many of them have side effects, much more than the simpler antibiotics.

Newer surgical techniques are being carried out. The very fact that these new techniques are being abandoned quickly shows that they had not been assessed fully before being put to use.

Many of these newer surgical procedures are so costly the people cannot afford them. They are told by the doctor that such operations are essential.

> The patient agrees to it, even though he/she cannot afford it. *Statesman*, Calcutta, 30 January 1991: A young man underwent open heart surgery. The cost originally estimated at Rs. 95,000 (under a poor patient scheme) came to about Rs. 1.5 lakhs. He has been missing. The family has lodged complaints with the police of "wrongful confinement' by the hospital for inability to pay the dues, estimated at Rs. 63,000 over and above the original estimate.

The competition between providers of medical care is becoming severe in the larger cities. Sometimes whole groups of professional and technical people are shifted, increasing the cost to the patient.

> *Business Standard,* Calcutta, 15 June, 1991 : "Col......... on the other hand, claims that the thirty doctors employed by the BMBHRC and a host of visiting doctors are among the best in the business.
>
> "Take Dr........... for example, we know he is the best and we lifted his whole team, including the nurses, from................ hospital, London".

A major problem with surgical technologies is their unnecessary use. There is an increasing realization that there is need to reduce the large number of surgical interventions, such as cesarian sections, hysterectomies and others, just as a reduction has occurred in the number of appendicectomies and tonsillectomies. Other costly curative technologies include lithotripsy for renal and gallstones, hemodialysis and coronary angioplasty.

An evaluative study of modem obstetrics from Vienna has shown that far too many unnecessary cesarian sections are being carried out. It has also shown that electronic monitoring has no advantage over the use of the stethoscope and may actually lead to unnecessary intervention.

There have been complaints that cesarian sections are being carried out, atleast occasionally for the convenience of the attending doctor and sometimes for monetary gains.

Preventive Technology

These include vaccines (newer ones, improvements in the production, storage, distribution and administration including the timings and number of times), safety measures in the industry, home, roads and elsewhere, prevention of pollution of air and water, use of iodized salts, oral rehydration in preventing dehydration and many others. These are welcome technologies that are cost-effective and bring benefits to all. Improvements in water supply and sanitation bring about better health. Unfortunately, not enough attention is paid to them. Even highly cost-effective vaccines are not available to the extent needed.

Rehabilitative Technology

Rehabilitative care has been the Cinderella of health care. There is increasing realization of the need of rehabilitation of the disabled, whatever be the type of disability. These technologies range from the simple aids to the highly sophisticated.

Technological advances in rehabilitation can be used in:

- prevention of disabilities,
- developing the inherent capabilities of the disabled,
- manufacture and fabrication of aids and appliances, and
- bringing about changes in the environment.

OTHER TECHNOLOGIES

Many other technologies can affect health. Among them will be those which help in creating health awareness, leading to health action. Improved technologies for health education and communication can help. There are technologies which promote health indirectly: Agriculture, education and improvement in environment, including better housing. Technologies can do the opposite also: Indiscriminate use of insecticides, pesticides and many other chemicals.

Choice: There are choices based on the system of values.

- Should the doctor use any and every technological tool to handle the particular problems of the sick?
- Should the doctor help nature to take its course and resort to technologies to help nature?

One consultant might claim that he has the clinical freedom to treat his patients with the newest and expensive technology or drug. At the same time there is responsibility to use carefully scarce resources. *Clinical freedom is freedom to do good; it carries responsibilities which must not be abused.*

ETHICAL CONSIDERATIONS

Several questions must be raised while considering adoption of a particular medical technology.

- Is this technology indicated? Is it necessary?
- What are the benefits? Does it improve patient outcome?
- Does it bring about better health? Does it increase wellness of the people, reduce morbidity, alleviate pain and improve the quality of life?

- What are the risks involved? What is the benefit: risk ratio?
- What is the cost? What is the burden on the individual, the family and the society?
- Is there a better alternative ? What are the other alternatives available?
- Can a cheaper alternative be used equally well? Is it cost-effective?

Doctor Diagnostic Centre Relationship

Many diagnostic centers have been springing up haphazardly. The costly equipment is often underutilized because the *real demand is small.* An artificial demand is built up. Sometimes "incentives" are offered to doctors for ordering these investigations. Ordering unnecessary investigations and investigations of doubtful value in the given circumstances is unethical.

Use of Equipment

There is a growing tendency to purchase sophisticated equipment. It is often a prestige issue. There is a tendency to apply expensive technology too soon, before it is properly evaluated for safety, efficacy and cost. Be careful in the purchase of equipment. Exercise care to ensure that we spend the scarce resources wisely. Do not buy equipment that is:

- inappropriate for the level of functioning,
- not cost-effective, and
- presented to the market place without adequate evaluation.

With the high speed of innovation, competition and aggressive marketing, newer equipment is marketed too quickly. There is early obsolescence.

Many a time sophisticated equipment is purchased, without adequate service backup. The result is that the costly equipment lies idle. It has been estimated that at any given time, *more than 30% of the sophisticated equipment in the country is out of use.* Palmer says in the "Epidemic of Investigations" in the *International Joumal of Epidemiology,* Vol 14: "Most of the imaging equipment currently used in small hospitals worldwide (when it works, which is not often) is excessive when related to the clinical needs and complex to operate and maintain".

The doctor has a duty to see that only such equipment as are necessary and can be used regularly are ordered for. The down time of the equipment should be as short as possible. The doctor who wants a particular equipment to be purchased has the responsibility to ensure that it works. The aspirations of the specialist (understandable as it is) must be tempered by the realities of the finance, usefulness and backup services.

Product Failure

There is not only early obsolescence. Failure rate is very high because the products are brought into the market too early because of excessive competition.

> Economic Times, Bombay, June 1, 1991: It has been a charmed half decade for St Jude Medical, Inc. The St Paul (Minn) maker of the world's most popular heart valve soared to the top of its lucrative market after two of its toughest rivals Baxter International Inc., and Pfizer Inc stopped selling their designs because of celebrated product failures. That let St Jude raise prices up to 10% annually without investing a dime to change its 14-year-old design. Last year, its profits surged 24%".

Appropriate Technology

There is a popular misconception among doctors when the term "appropriate technology" is used. Appropriate technology is neither unscientific nor is it a returning to primitive traditions. Appropriateness depends on the particular need and situation.

Appropriate technology is:
- scientifically effective,
- culturally acceptable,
- economic, and
- adapted to local skills and knowledge.

Appropriate technology is sensitive to the environment and does not spoil it. It takes into consideration the available technical know-how so that proper use and maintenance are taken care of.

Assessment of Healthcare Technologies

Newer technologies coming up all the time need assessment, before they are adopted. Such assessment should be carried out by independent committees consisting of experts from various disciplines—healthcare professionals, technologists, economists, administrators and others. The participants should not have conflicts of interest. Technical and economic appraisals must be carried out on all new medical technologies. The criteria would include:

- efficiency and effectiveness;
- quality of the process of care;
- use of human resources, scientific, professional and technical;
- use of financial resources, capital and recurring;
- ethics of resource allocation.

Medical Technology and the Family

All technology affects the family; medical technology more so. They do so in varying degrees. Among the technologies affecting the family, the most important are the reproductive technologies. They have the greatest impact on the values of family living.

Medical Care as a Business

It is often thought that the private sector may be allowed to setup the centers for sophisticated high technology, if they so wish as only private funds are involved. This is not so. Public funds are involved. Financial institutions give loans and advances at subsidised rates to import the equipment and establish the high technology medical care centers. Foreign currency is made available. Often customs duty exemptions, amounting to large amounts are given. It has been estimated that the promoter's cost is often reduced to about 10% of the project cost.

Medicine has become big business. Most of the big business houses have moved into "medical care". There is a change in the perception of the goals of medical care. Are these newer activities aimed at improving the quality of life or at maximizing profit, with high returns on the investment? Are the ideas of what people consider as good quality of life being manipulated to serve the financial interests of the corporations newly come into the medical field?

CHAPTER 17 Alternate Medicine

There is growing interest in alternative medicine. There is a certain amount of dissatisfaction or disillusionment with 'modern medicine' because:

- 'modern'medicine does not give cure or even relief in many instances,
- it is often very expensive, beyond the affordability of many patients,
- some people consider that it can be hazardous because it is not 'natural', and
- of other reasons.

There are many systems in vogue in India. Some are time honored remedies. Many of them might be able to render help, if practised correctly. They often have a holistic approach. Unfortunately charlatans and get-rich-quick merchants of medical care play up on the fears and emotions of the patients (and their relatives).

They may cause more harm than good. There is a rising tide of quackery. Untrained and unqualified persons often claim to be practitioners of alternative medicine.

There is need for assessing the value of alternative therapy. The methodology for their assessment may be different from the 'scientific' methods adopted for 'modern' medicine. But evaluation is a must. This must be done with a healthy respect to these therapies.

It is also necessary to insist on certain standards and qualifications of the practitioners of alternative medicine. While there are recognized institutions giving training in some systems, there is no such training for other systems. There might be some informal training.

Sometimes dangerous and inappropriate drugs are promoted and used. Media is used to advertise these drugs. People who have only an imperfect understanding of the virtues and vices of drugs are tempted to try these drugs. The patient is often a prey to plausible suggestions.

There is an increasing tendency among practitioners of 'modern' medicine to prescribe drugs found in the materia medica of other systems or even those which are not found in them just because they are advertised widely with all kinds of claims. Prescribing some Ayurvedic medicines along with other drugs is becoming quite popular. Misuse of drugs and procedures by persons unqualified in those systems may add to rather than subtract from the patient's problems. So also some of the practitioners of other systems use indiscriminately some of the medicines found in 'modern medicine' pharmacopoeias with often adverse results.

There have been many moves for the study of integrated system of medicine but they cannot be said to have been very successful. Such efforts are continuing. There are many courses of studies in integrated medicine.

The National Health Policy (1982) states : "The country has a large stock of health manpower, comprising private practitioners in various systems, for example, *Ayurveda, Unani, Siddha, Yoga, Homeopathy, Naturopathy,* etc. This resource has not so far been adequately used".

The Government of India is keen on promoting Indian systems of medicine. They are "widely used by all classes of people and felt to be a central part of the cultural heritage. Yet the knowledge and ethics of its practitioners are said to have declined from those of former times. In some respects an irregular medical practice and in other respects part of the regular medical system, the modernization of Ayurvedic and Arabic medicine in India brings them into an ambiguous paramedical relationship to modern scientific medicine"—Charles Leslie, 1974.

Ethical problems can arise in the relationships between practitioners of modern medicine and the practitioners of other systems of medicine.

OTHER SYSTEMS OF MEDICINE

Health care in India uses many systems of medicine. There are practitioners of different systems practising side by side. The Indian Systems of Medicine include Ayurveda, Siddha, Unani,

Naturopathy and Yoga. Homeopathy is also very popular. There are about 4.91 lakh registered practitioners of Indian Systems of Medicine and Homeopathy (1990–91). They enjoy high acceptance and respect of the people. There are two councils, viz. the Central Council of Indian Medicine and Central Council of Homeopathy which are responsible for regulating the practice of medical practitioners in the respective fields.

Ayurveda

The other system which had been in vogue from ancient times and continues to be practised on a large scale even today is Ayurveda, the Science of life. The collected writings of Charaka, Susruta, Bhela, Kasyapa and others give the philosophical basis, principles and practice of Ayurveda. According to Ayurveda, there must be equilibrium of three doshas, *Vayu, Pitta and Kapha*. Ayurveda has eight divisions including surgery; surgery itself has eight subdivisions but the practice of surgery by Ayurvedic physicians declined later on.

The ancient Ayurvedic system influenced by the teachings of *the Upanishads,* treated man as whole—body, mind and what was beyond mind.

Ayurveda places great emphasis on ethics. All the teachers of Ayurveda gave detailed instructions for the proper behavior of the medical student and the practising doctor. The student, the teacher and the doctor on the threshold of practice had to take pledges of ethical conduct.

The training in Ayurveda may be various types: Suddha (pure) Ayurveda, Ayurveda integrated with varying amounts of modern medicine and non-formal training including apprenticeship to Ayurvedic physicians.

Unani

Unani medicine as practised today is a hybrid between the Greco Arab and Ayurvedic medicine. The Unani physician (*Hakim*) has his own code of conduct, closely allied to the code propounded by Hippocrates. Unani practice which started with the coming of the Arabs, flourished during the Mughul rule. It continues to be practised actively even now.

Siddha

Siddha medicine is practised mainly in Tamil Nadu. Its origin is probably in the Dravidian culture and then it absorbed Ayurveda. There was also the Arab influence. The treatment is by means of herbal and mineral substances.

Homeopathy

This is a system of therapy, first propounded by Dr Samuel Hahneman. There is a vital force which is the essence of all life. It is necessary to maintain the vital force in a healthy state. There are certain basic principles of homeopathy:

- law of similars—a drug capable of producing certain symptoms in health will produce cure of the disease with the same set of symptoms.
- use the minimum dose required to effect cure.
- use, as far as possible, a single remedy which fits with the pattern of disease.

Naturopathy

This is a promotive and preventive form of therapy. There is natural body resistance and all that is needed is to support it. Even when there is illness, no medicine is given. Disease is considered as the body's effort to cleanse itself of the impurities which have accumulated in the body. The cure is effected through the elements of nature (air, water, earth and the rays of sun).

Water is considered as very important. The ideal intake of water is considered to be about four liters per day. Plain water is taken on rising, at midmorning, half an hour before lunch, midafternoon, evening and at bedtime. Other fluids can also be taken.

It is important to eat the right kind of food. Each season produces its own kind of fruits and vegetables. These are considered to be related to body needs at that time. Fruits and vegetables are preferably eaten raw. The diet is important when the person is ill. Diet may be of three types: Soothing, eliminative and constructive. Non-vegetarian dishes, pickles, condiments, alcohol, coffee and tea are prohibited in naturopathy.

Fasting is considered good medicine. Accumulation of toxic matter in the digestive system is thought to be the root cause of many disease. It is necessary to clean the digestive tract. Fasting helps in the process. The patient may take water, lime juice or fruit juices, depending on the condition of the patient and nature of the disease.

Enema is commonly used. It cleans the lower bowel. Plain water is used. Cold enema is given for inflammatory conditions of the colon, especially in dysentery, ulcerative colitis and other diarrheal conditions. Hot enema is used to relieve irritation. Water prepared with neem leaves is recommended in amebiasis and worm infestations.

Hot foot bath is recommended. Keep feet and legs in a tub filled with water at a temperature of 40–45°C. Cover with a blanket. Keep for 10–20 minutes. Wash with cold water.

Mud therapy: Keep soaked mud, collected from river banks and cleaned of stones and dirty particles in thin muslin cloth above the patient's abdomen. Mud bath can be applied to the whole body and then exposed to sunlight for 20–30 minutes or until the mud gets dry.

Heliotherapy (sun bath) may be taken directly between 8 AM to 11 AM and 2 PM to 4 PM in winter and between 7 AM to 9 AM and 3 PM to 5 PM in summer.

Herbal Medicine

Many people turn to herbs. The term *herbal* brings up visions of something natural, something healing. Many of them are found in folk medicine and are effective. Most of them do no harm. Many of them are familiar ones, like ginger, garlic, tamarind, clove, asafoetida, etc. But some of the herbal medicines can be harmful. They can produce toxicity, hypotension, liver damage, etc. There is need to differentiate between the useful, harmless and harmful remedies. The plants have to be identified carefully, as mistakes can easily occur.

Ayurvedic texts describe contraindications, sideeffects and adverse effects of the use of some plants and their preparations. Some are contraindicated in children; others in the elderly; still others in pregnant or lactating mothers.

Drugless Therapies

These therapies are other than surgery, ECT and other procedures used in modern medical practice.

Management of patients is complex. Many procedures may bring healing and one such method is by the use of drugs, or chemical substances with certain properties. In drugless therapies, drugs are not used for treatment.

Yoga

Yoga is used for disciplining mind and body. It is not a system of medicine but a way of living in health. There are a number of ways of doing it. The most important text is the *Yogasutra* of Patanjali (2nd century BC). According to this, there are eight steps to perfection.

1. Yama
2. Niyama
3. Asana
4. Pranayama
5. Prathyahara
6. Dharana
7. Dhyana
8. Samadhi

The best known are the *asanas* or postures. Yoga helps to improve bodily strength, endurance and cardiorespiratory functions. Some of the *asanas (e.g. savasana)* are useful in bringing down high blood pressure; others help in improving circulation; still others improve respiration.

Massage

This is used for many therapeutic purposes including improvement of circulation to a particular part. Massage may be done by hand or other equipment. When done by hand, there is body contact.

Massage is a common form of treatment in Ayurveda. But, in Ayurveda, medicated oils are used and hence it is a form of drug therapy.

Acupuncture

It emanated as a system of treatment in China. The earliest references to the use of Acupuncture are found in the Yellow Emperor's Manual in Corporeal Medicine (200 BC). It is practised side by side with modern medicine. Needles are used to puncture the skin. According to the traditional Chinese theory, there are hypothetical channels through which Qi (the invisible life force) flows. Each of these channels or meridians is linked to the activity of an organ or organ system of the body. Points on each meridian can be stimulated to produce balance and remove imbalance or dysfunction. Acupuncture is used to relieve pain, relax muscles, release hormones and endorphin, raise the immunity level, and for the treatment of common diseases. Relief from mental depression may also be effected. Electrical stimulation through the needles is also used.

Acupressure: This method is similar to acupuncture. Pressure is exerted instead of sticking needles. Pressure is exerted mainly in the palms and soles of feet. Different points are said to be present for different organs and structures in the body.

Shiatsu : This is the Japanese system based on principles similar to acupuncture. It uses pressure with the fingers at acupuncture points.

Magnetotherapy

This system utilizes magnets or electromagnetic fields to influence the vital force in the body. Magnetic waves are presumed to act on the cell and change the potentials. Any imbalance in the magnetic field in any organ may result in a pathological state. The external application of a magnetic field produces changes in the charged particles. It can improve circulation and alter the permeability. Magnetotherapy is said to bring about quicker healing of wounds, ulcers and fractures.

Other forms of drugless therapies include manipulative therapy, hypnotherapy, osteopathy, chiropractic, reflexology, counseling, psychotherapy and biofeedback.

It is important to realize that these therapies (some old; some new) may have something to offer in the care and cure of the patient. It is unethical to:

- condemn them saying that we do not have scientific proof of their efficacy, and
- use them without knowing how to use them.

Cross Practice

The law of the land restricts the practice of medicine to that system of medicine in which the practitioner is qualified (trained) and registered under the appropriate council. The Supreme Court, in Ashwin Patel-*vs*-Poonam Verma, decided that practising any type of medicine without the requisite knowledge and qualification would amount to 'negligence per se' and described it as quackary (Supreme Court decision, 1998). This prompted some Food and Drugs Authorities to issue orders preventing chemists from selling allopathic drugs when prescribed by non-allopathic doctors. To counter this, some State Governments issued notifications under the Drugs and Cosmetics Act (section 2) permitting the use of allopathic medicines by non-allopathic medical graduates.

Cross practice can pose dangers:

> "A 62 year-old man was brought into the casualty at KEM Hospital (Mumbai) in an unconscious state. When questioned by doctors, his relatives revealed that he was a diabetic whose hyperglycemia was well-controlled with insulin and glibenclamide. Five days earlier, he had been started on an Ayurvedic drug for psoriasis. He developed giddiness following ingestion of the drug but ignored it. Subsequently he became unconscious. He succumbed to hypoglycemic coma".
>
> —Issues in Medical Ethics, 5 (3): 94, 1997

Many issues arise. Most of the rural population have to depend on non-allopathic doctors for their health needs. People have to go to non-allopathic doctors for injuries, snake-bite, etc. for which the particular non-allopathic discipline may not have effective therapy. Will preventing the non-allopathic doctor from administering the particular drug (because it is not included in their curriculum) amount to depriving a patient of essential health care? Sometimes, allopathic medicine may not have a therapy against a particular disease. Should the doctor encourage the patient to go to a practitioner of alternate system of medicine? Should allopathic treatment be combined while the patient is taking treatment (for another condition) from a practitioner of other systems of medicine?

CHAPTER 18

Organ Transplantation

In 1831, Jeremy Bentham asked a question: "Of what use is a dead man to the living"? He had autopsies in view. But today many organs are taken from the dead person to be transplanted into the living, prolonging life or giving relief.

Many organs and tissues are being transplanted. These include:

1. regenerative tissues, such as blood and bone marrow. The donated blood is replaced soon by the body of the healthy donor and it is easy to perform. Bone marrow transplantation is much more difficult,
2. paired organs, such as kidney. The remaining kidney is able to carry out the functions,
3. non-paired organs, essential for life (e.g. heart),
4. fetal tissues (e.g. parts of brain).

The organs and tissues may be obtained from living persons (where compatible with life) or from cadavers (cornea, kidney, lung, heart, liver, pancreas, etc.). The demand for organs is on the increase. The available organs are unable to meet the demands. The methods used to meet the demands raise many ethical issues.

LIVE DONORS

In the case of some transplants, close relatives may donate one of their paired organ like kidney for truly altruistic reasons. Even when the donation is apparently altruistic, there can be many hidden factors. There may be inducements and social, psychological and other pressures.

The large majority of live donors in India are the poor. They do so for monetary gain. There is commercialization with trafficking in organs. People are treated as a source of organs for sale and purchase as any other commodity. The economic situation of the poor is exploited. The rich patients (Indian and foreign) are prepared to pay. An axis is formed with agents scouting for the poor donors, especially villagers and slum dwellers, offering them some money. The larger share of the amounts is pocketed by the agents, the doctors and the hospitals. A few doctors have raised their voice against this unethical trafficking in organs but many others are not bothered and carry on the 'trade".

"Mentally retarded brother to donate kidney today"

—The New Indian Express, Bangalore, March 12, 1999

VNP is a deaf-mute mentally retarded person. His brother VNS is the sole bread winner of the family consisting of his mother, brother, wife and a child. He needs a kidney transplant. The mother gives her consent but the would be 'donor' does not give the consent nor object to it. Is it ethical to transplant the kidney under the circumstances?

Can human organs be treated just like any other property owned by the person? Will the laws applicable to transfer of "goods" (Sale of Goods Act, 1930 and Transfer of Property Act, 1982) be applicable to transfer of human organs? Will there be an enforceable contract ? Does the transfer of human organ go counter to public policy? As a social aspect, we find it difficult to accept the human organ on par with other goods.

The question is asked; if blood can be sold for a consideration (as happens in commercial blood banks), why not other organs also? Blood is a tissue which is replaced easily; it is regenerated fully. Free, voluntary donation of blood by healthy donors is to be encouraged. Its sale and commercialization, though accepted by society at present are to be replaced by free donation.

"Payment for organs and tissues for transplantation should be prohibited. A financial incentive compromises the voluntariness of the choice and the altruistic basis of organ and tissue donation—organs suspected to have been obtained through commercial transactions should not be accepted for transplantation".

—World Medical Association, 52nd General Assembly, Edinburgh, Oct, 2000

CADAVER DONATION

Most of the organ transplants in other countries are organs obtained from cadavers. The organs must be removed at the earliest. Death is a process. Different tissues and cells die at different times. Because of the need for early removal before the particular tissue dies, determination of the moment of death is very important. If we wait for the removal of tissues after the complete cessation of heart beat and respiration, the tissues and organs may be irreversably dead and become useless.

Countries are defining death as "brain death", where irreversible changes occur in the brainstem and there is no likelihood of the person surviving. Electroencephalographic and other changes occur. Such instances can occur often enough in road and other accidents. The organs can be kept in reasonably good shape by artificial perfusion and ventilation. Where the law permits, organs can be removed quickly to be transplanted into waiting patients. The demand being very high and there being urgency, we have to be careful in deciding the moment of brain death. The transplant surgeon would like to get the organ as early as possible. To avoid misuse, it is suggested that there should be two independent teams, a patient care team and a transplant team. The patient care team will ensure the patient's interest.

Even in such cases, the relatives may not be agreeable for the removal of the organs. There are people who consider the inviolability of the human body even in death. The Confucian Book of Filial Piety speaks of keeping the dead body in tact. It is necessary to have the consent of the person, given prior to death, or of the closest relatives agreeing to the procedures of removal of the organ.

WHAT IS BRAIN DEATH ?

A person is said to be brain dead when the brain is so severely damaged by injury, loss of blood supply or disease that recovery is impossible, although the heart may be kept beating and the lungs working with artificial support. In the brain dead, we have what is described as "heart beating cadaver" or "ventilated corpse".

Guideline for Diagnosis of Brain Death

1. Establish a cause capable of bringing about brain death.
2. Exclude all potentially reversible conditions like drug intoxication, metabolic and endocrine disorders, hypothermia and neuromuscular paralysis by drugs or disease.
3. Patient is in deep coma and shows no response within the cranial nerve distribution to stimulation applied to any part of the body.
4. Absence of brainstem reflexes, such as pupillary, corneal and vestibulo-ocular.
5. Patient makes no respiratory effort when taken off the respirator for 10 minutes.
6. The electroencephalogram is flat.

The above conditions must persist when the person is re-assessed after an interval of more than 6 hours. Children below 3 years of age are excluded.

ETHICAL ISSUES IN TRANSPLANTATION

Many ethical issues arise:

1. Setting up a transplant unit is *very expensive.* A liver transplant unit may cost anything upwards of a crore of Rupees. Each transplant may cost more than one lakh of Rupees. The resources (money, men and materials) could be used more efficiently for primary health care, benefitting many times the number of people.
2. The *focus* of the institution/organization comes on to the transplant program. Other departments are upgraded to support the transplant unit with less attention to other activities.
3. There are *human costs.* Patients and relatives suffer emotionally waiting for an organ to become available. Half the patients die while waiting for a suitable organ.
4. *Commercialization and unethical practices* in procuring organs.
5. The *choice of the recipient is* difficult. Who will decide as to who is to receive the transplant from among those waiting? The most ill? The most needy? The person with the best possible results? First come, first-served? Influence? Money?

The United States of America has the *Uniform Anatomical Gift Act.*

Uniform Anatomical Gift Act, USA

The Act provides for:

1. Any individual of sound mind and eighteen years of age or more may give all or any part of his body..... the gift to take effect upon death.
2. In the absence of a gift by the deceased, and of any objection by the deceased, his or her relatives, in a stated order of priority: Spouse, adult children, parents, adult brothers and sisters, etc., have the power to give the body or any of its contents.
3. The recipient of a gift is restricted to hospitals, doctors, medical and dental schools, universities, tissue banks and a specified individual in need of treatment. The purposes are restricted to transplantation therapy, research, education and the advancement of medical or dental science.
4. A gift may be made by will (to be effective immediately upon death without waiting for probate) or by a card or other document. If the donor is too sick or incapable of signing, it can be signed for him if two witnesses are present. A gift made by a relative can be made by documents or by telegraph or a recorded telephone message or other recorded message.
5. A gift may be revoked at anytime.
6. A donee may accept or reject a gift.

The Act gives blanket protection against law suits and criminal proceedings to any person "who acts in good faith in accordance with the terms of this Act".

The Act deals with dead bodies only. It does not regulate gifts of body materials by living persons.

The Council of Europe has made a more radical legal code which regulates tissue or organ removal both from the dead and living person. It extends to all tissues, except embryos, ovaries, ova, testes and sperm.

In July 1989, the *Human Organ Transplant Act was* enacted in UK. This was mainly in response to a hue and cry raised on report of donors from Turkey and India being induced to sell their kidney to wealthy recipients in UK.

Fetal Tissue

Fetal tissues are being transplanted. Persons suffering from Parkinsonism are supposed to benefit from the transplants of fetal brain. This is expected to give the deficient neurotransmitter. It is now observed that the beneficial effects of such transplants are not sustained. But use of fetal tissues raises many ethical issues. Women may be willing to conceive to produce and grow fetuses which will then be "harvested" for monetary considerations, to give the fetal tissues for various purposes including transplant of tissues.

The United States Government, in 1989, rejected the request for support for research in fetal tissue transplantation for Parkinsonism and diabetes mellitus because of the ethical issues involved.

WHO Guiding Principles on Human Organ Transplantation (as endorsed by the Forty-fourth World Health Assembly, 1991)

Organs and tissues (referred to in this text as "organs") may be removed from the bodies of deceased and living persons for the purpose of transplantation only in accordance with the following Guiding Principles.

Organs may be removed from the bodies of deceased persons for the purpose of transplantation if:

a. any consents required by law are obtained and
b. there is no reason to believe that the deceased person objected to such removal, in the absence of any formal consent given during the person's lifetime.
   - Physicians determining that the death of a potential donor has occurred should not be directly involved in organ removal from the donor and subsequent transplantation procedures, or be responsible for the care of potential recipients of such organs.
   - Organs for transplantation should be removed preferably from the bodies of deceased persons. However, adult living persons may donate organs, but in general such donors should be genetically related to the recipients. Exceptions may be made in the case of transplantation of bone marrow and other acceptable regenerative tissues.
   - An organ may be removed from the body of an adult living donor for the purpose of transplantation if the donor gives free consent. The donor should be free of any undue influ-

ence and pressure and sufficiently informed to be able to understand and weigh the risks, benefits and consequences of consent.

- No organ should be removed from the body of a living minor for the purpose of transplantation. Exceptions may be made under national law in the case of regenerative tissues.
- The human body and its parts cannot be the subject of commercial transactions. Accordingly, giving or receiving payment (including any other compensation or reward) for organs should be prohibited.
- Advertising the need for or availability of organs with a view to offering or seeking payment should be prohibited.
- It should be prohibited for physicians and other health professionals to engage in organ transplantation procedures if they have reason to believe that the organs concerned have been the subject of commercial transactions.
- It should be prohibited for any person or facility involved in organ transplantation procedures to receive any payment that exceeds a justifiable fee for the services rendered.
- In the light of the principles of distributive justice and equity, donated organs should be made available to patients on the basis of medical need and not on the basis of financial or other considerations.
- "Human organs" used here do not include reproductive tissues embryos, ovaries, testes, ova and spermatozoa.

The Transplantation of Human Organs Act, 1994

The Government of India enacted a law "to provide for the regulation of removal, storage and transplantation of human organs for therapeutic purposes and for the prevention of commercial dealings in human organs and for matters connected therewith or incident thereto". The rules thereunder were published in the Gazette of India in February, 1995. In spite of this, the exploitation of the poor to part with their organs (particularly kidneys) continued.

"**Kidney transplant: COD probe on**

After dragging its feet for as long as it could, the Appropriate Authority which monitors the implementation of the Transplantation of Human Organs (THO) Act 1994, has finally given the green signal to the Corps of Detectives (COD) to investigate the large scale clearance of 1,016 unrelated kidney transplants from 1995 to December 2001 in major transplant centers in the state.

Sources told *The Hindu* that COD would now investigate the clearance for transplants along with the January 15 scandal in Mandya's Holalu village, where nine agents "pursuaded" 36 villagers to sell their kidneys for paltry sums. The attempt would be to break the transplant centre - official - agent nexus which had made commerce in kidneys possible".

—The Hindu, Bangalore, 6.6.2002

The law provides the Authority certain functions and responsibilities. These include:

1. periodic inspection of the hospitals (approved for transplantation);
2. suspend or cancel registration of transplant centres violating the law;
3. enforce standards for hospitals; and
4. investigate any complaint of breach of the provisions of the Act.

Ethical Considerations

The buying and selling of human organs have been considered unethical and immoral traditionally.

"In a Resolution on Physicians' Conduct concerning Human Organ Transplantation adopted at the 46th WMA General Assembly in Stockholm in September 1994, the professional body recorded "significant concern" over growing reports of physicians participating in the transplantation of human organs or tissue taken from the cadavers of executed prisoners or handicapped persons (whose deaths were "believed to have been expedited to facilitate the harvesting of their organs") or "the bodies of poor people who have agreed to part with their organs for commercial purposes" or"the bodies of children kidnapped for this purpose". Declaring the participation of physicians in such practices to be in "direct contravention" of the 1987 guidelines, WMA called upon all national medical associations to uphold these guidelines and asked for severe disciplining of the physicians involved in cases of "infraction".

—Frontline, April 12, 2002

CHAPTER 19

HIV/AIDS

Acquired immunodeficiency syndrome (AIDS) is the modern scourge. It is a pandemic affecting all the continents. India has a huge number of people infected by the human immunodeficiency virus (HIV). They will end up as fatal AIDS patients. The estimate based on HIV Sentinel Surveillance for the year 2001 is 3.31 million HIV infections in the adult population (15–49 years age group). Taking into consideration, the unaccounted groups, such as other age groups and intravenous drug users, the total estimate (additional 20%) comes to 3.97 million HIV infected persons in India in the year 2001. The estimates for 1998, 1999 and 2000 of HIV infections were 3.5 millions, 3.7 millions and 3.86 millions, respectively. Though there is increase in the absolute numbers of those infected, the rate of increase seems to be slowing down. The incidence of fresh infections seems to be getting reduced.

There is no known cure. There are a number of antiretroviral agents which can reduce the rate of progress of the disease and be useful for certain interventions. Regimes of multidrug therapies have been worked out. They are in use in the affluent countries. They are not easily available for the poorer sections of the society because of the prohibitive cost. The medicines have to be continued as long as the patients live. Further, the investigations to monitor the progress of the disease and adjust the treatment are expensive. India and some other countries are in a position to produce relatively cheaper drugs. But these countries are not allowed to market such drugs in other countries because of the new patent restrictions (regulations by the World Trade Organization). Tens of thousands of people die while the debate on the rights of pharmaceutical firms continues.

There is also no effective vaccine, though attempts at developing vaccines and their trial are going on. Such a situation of lack of preventive and curative medicine is a situation which leads to many spurious claims. The gullible public fall victims to such claims.

Human immunodeficiency virus causes diseases by itself but more importantly allows opportunistic infections. The body is unable to defend against such infections. The Centre for Diseases Control, Atlanta, USA, has listed 27 such infections. Other conditions like Kaposi's sarcoma and non-Hodgkin's lymphomas occur. In Africa, AIDS is known as SLIM disease, because of wasting and significant weight loss. In India, an HIV infected person is said to have AIDS, if there is:

- prolonged fever,
- loss of weight,
- diarrhea,
- cough, and
- suppressed immune status as shown by lowered counts of T4 lymphocytes.

Most of the patients have tuberculosis, both pulmonary and extrapulmonary. There may be gastroenteritis.

TRANSMISSION OF HIV

The most common method of transmission is through sexual intercourse, heterosexual or homosexual. There are certain groups with high-risk behavior, such as commercial sex workers. The likelihood of getting infected is much greater, when there are many sexual partners. The best policy is to stay with the married partner only. Encouraging social and moral values against promiscuity and discouraging prostitution can bring on large dividends.

Another mode of transmission is through blood and blood products. Infected blood or blood products, if transfused, could infect the recipient very easily. Much of the world's blood is bought and sold like any other commodity. The professional donors live in poor conditions and poor health. Many of these professional donors are infected with HIV and hence rate of transmission is high. When detected the professional donor moves off to another region and continues to donate blood. Testing of blood donors for HIV is mandatory. This has produced another problem. Even voluntary donors are reluctant to come forward to donate blood because they know that their blood will be tested and fear the test result. There is need to have rational use of blood. Blood should be used only when really needed. In such instances, blood should be made available from voluntary healthy donors.

Needles and syringes contaminated with infected blood can transmit the infection. This occurs commonly in intravenous drug abusers who share needles. This is a major method of transmission among drug abusers in the *north-eastern* parts of India. Such transmission can occur in health care also, if the needles and syringes are not properly sterilized. Where possible, disposable needles and syringes may be used. Disposing of the disposable needles and syringes should be done carefully.

Transmission can occur from mother to baby (fetus) in the womb. The virus can cross the placenta and infect the baby. Infection can also occur during childbirth. This is less common and is due to infection through the secretions. Infection can be passed on to the baby during breastfeeding.

HIV ANTIBODY TESTING

AIDS is the final stage of infection with HIV. It can take many years before an infected person develops signs and symptoms of AIDS. Meanwhile, the virus may be passed on to others unknowingly.

We can detect the presence of antibodies to HIV usually within a few weeks. The period when we cannot detect the antibodies, even when infected by HIV is known as the "window period". Transmission of virus can occur during this period.

The test for HIV antibody must satisfy two criteria:

1. Sensitivity: The test result will be positive when antibodies to HIV are present.
2. Specificity: The result will be negative if antibodies to HIV are not present.

An ideal test will have 100% sensitivity and 100% specificity. But no test is ideal.

Objectives of HIV Testing

There are three main objectives:

1. Diagnosis of HIV infection in individuals. Testing is done for prevention of transmission and care. The test is also done in antenatal clinics.

2. Screening of donated blood for blood safety. Such testing is mandatory. It is a highly cost-effective preventive measure. Blood transfusion has almost 100% efficiency in transmission; hence testing and control are important.
3. Epidemiological surveillance of HIV prevalence.

Types of Tests

The most widely used test is the enzyme linked immunosorbent assay (ELISA). The ELISA test is suitable for batch testing: 96 to several hundred specimens can be tested per day. It requires costly equipment, maintenance and trained personnel. It also takes time for the results to be known.

There are also simple, rapid tests:

- agglutination tests,
- immunocomb tests,
- immunodot tests, using flow through membranes,
- immunochromatographic membrane tests.

These tests are available in kit forms. The procedures are easy; there are less chances of error. The results can be obtained within a few minutes. The tests can be designed as a single test or in multiple format with a limited number of specimens. The test kits do not require refrigeration and can be stored at temperatures between 2 and 30°C. They rank high in specificity, reliability and reproducibility and are cost-effective.

Open heart surgery was performed in a private hospital. Three bottles of blood tested for HIV, were available. But, during the operation, one more bottle of blood was required most urgently. One more bottle of blood was obtained; there was no time to wait for the result of the ELISA test. The blood was transfused as a life-saving measure. The mother and her later offspirng became HIV positive.

Was it ethical to have transfused the untested blood? Could the situation have been avoided, if rapid test was available?

Mandatory HIV Testing

There are people who advocate mandatory (without consent) testing, following a more aggressive path in finding out who is infected with HIV with the intention to protect society. Is this acceptable? The answer, at present, is a firm 'no', because

- there is stigma and the person will suffer exclusion and discrimination;
- the person can have a reasonable productive life, as the disease AIDS develops only after some years after infection;
- making HIV testing mandatory is a coercive act;
- no cure is available at present, though we can prolong life with antiretroviral therapy;
- infection with HIV is for life; and
- the infection is not contagious, unlike other infectious diseases, such as tuberculosis or typhoid.

HIV is spread mainly through sexual intercourse. To arrest the disease behavioral change is required. This cannot be achieved by mandatory testing. Reduction of spread may be obtained by creating awareness and counseling.

Some people advocate mandatory HIV testing of special groups:
- People with high-risk behavior, such as:
  - commercial sex workers;
  - long distance truck drivers;
  - intravenous drug users;
- Premarital, to prevent spread to the proposed spouse;
- Pregnant women as part of antenatal care. If the mother is found to be HIV positive, action can be taken to prevent vertical transmission to the offspring by treatment with antiviral agents.

Mandatory testing will not help in the above groups. Counseling followed by testing can help. We may have to reconsider the position when an effective cure becomes possible.

HIV Testing and Confidentiality

HIV testing should be done only with:
- informed consent;
- confidentiality; and
- counseling.

HIV Testing and Employment

The employer is interested in knowing the health status of the employee because the employer has to ensure that the employee:
- is capable of carrying out the job efficiently,
- is not a health hazard to other persons in the workplace, and

- is likely to continue to carryout the work for a reasonable period of employment.

The above objectives are likely to be achieved by pre-employment and periodical health check-ups. But in the case of HIV testing, the employer has no access to the result of the test because the testing is confidential.

Ordinarily, the HIV positive person is not a danger to the co-workers or others. But in certain situations, care must be exercised, e.g. a surgeon. The surgeon should be advised to keep away from performing operations. He/she should not come into contact with the blood of the patient (avoid mixing of blood).

In the case of health workers, there is the possibility of needle stick injury. This can cause transmission of infection, though such spread is rare. Postexposure prophylaxis can be resorted to in case of needle stick injuries.

HIV Infection and Marriage

HIV test results are confidential. But, in a case where the hospital came to know of the proposed marriage of an HIV positive person, the hospital informed the parent of the situation. A suit was filed against the hospital for breach of confidentiality. The Supreme Court decided that, as it involved transmission of an infection for which there was, at present, no cure, it was right to have disclosed the result of the test and thereby preventing marriage (threat to the life of the partner). By its September, 1998 judgement, the court suspended the right to marry of the HIV positive person and made it punishable under Sections 269 and 270 of the IPC.

Does the judgement infringe the human rights of the affected person? Will the position change if people take conscious decisions to marry the affected persons?

HIV Infection and Intravenous Drug Use

One of the modes of spread of HIV infection is by sharing contaminated needles during injection of drugs. Such spread can be prevented by:

- helping individuals to abstain from drug injection (relapses are common);
- accessing a needle exchange program;
- educating the person to clean the needle and syringe with bleach.

The last two alternatives are considered morally wrong as they will be promoting drug addiction but are justified as the lesser of the two evils.

Ethical Problems Connected with HIV Testing

- The testing should be done with proper informed consent. Such informed consent is also necessary to have pretest counseling.
- Testing on the request of a third party (Government, educational institutions and employers) is ethically questionable. It can violate privacy and autonomy.
- HIV testing is expensive. Extensive screening tests will be a drain on the resources. Such screening may not be beneficial.
- Information that the person is infected with HIV should be given only after the confirmatory test results. Often when the screening result comes as positive, the information is given. Confirmatory test may be negative. But by that time psychological and social problems might have been created.
- If a person has tested positive, there is need for postcounseling and psychosocial support. Even if the person has tested negative, counseling is necessary as the person may develop a false sense of security which can tempt the person to continue the risk behavior.
- An infected individual may remain apparently 'healthy'and able to carry on with his/her activities for many years. Denying the person such activities will not be correct. The person should be allowed to continue with his activities without unnecessary constraints.

HIV-1 and HIV-2

A practical problem is with respect to variants of HIV. A German researcher has found both types in blood samples collected from high-risk groups in Mumbai. Among the samples tested,

- 52% were found infected,
- 7% tested positive for HIV-2, and
- 15% showed double infection (HIV-1 and HIV-2)

  Other variants may occur.

Psychological Dimensions of HIV Testing

The initial reaction of most of the patients to the information that his/her blood is HIV positive is one of shock and disbelief. It leads to fear. He/she does not know where to turn for help. To whom can he/ she tell ? What is he/she going to do with his/her life ? The person may take to abuse of drugs or alcohol. Suicidal action may follow. The patient may become depressed. There is need for counseling, pre and post-test.

The family also goes through psychological stress. It affects the spouse maximally. But others also react to the news.

PREVENTION AND CONTROL OF HIV INFECTION

Legislation

Attempts have been made to have legislation aimed at preventing the spread of HIV infection.

The Goa Act on AIDS provided for the isolation of HIV infected persons. Guidelines had been issued by the Government of India for HIV screening of foreigners. It required HIV free certificate or compulsory HIV testing of foreigners intending to stay in India for more than 1 year. It also provided for deporting HIV positive foreigners.

The Government of India brought forward the Acquired Immunodeficiency Syndrome (AIDS) Prevention Bill 1989, Bill No. XX of 1989.

"To provide for the prevention and control of the spread of Human Immunodeficiency Virus (HIV) infection and to provide for specialised medical treatment and social support to, and rehabilitation of persons suffering from Acquired lmmunodeficiency Syndrome (AIDS) and for matters connected therewith and incidental thereto."

Objects and Reasons

AIDS has become a major health hazard. No vaccine is presently available. It is also not possible to cure the disease.

A surveillance program on AIDS was initiated in India in 1985. The long incubation period renders identification based on clinical symptoms alone inadequate. Surveillance based on serology is necessary to prevent spread of HIV which causes AIDS.

It is necessary to:
1. take effective measures to prevent the spread of HIV,
2. detect persons infected,
3. prevent transmission by them of infection to others,
4. provide counseling, health education and social support, and
5. rehabilitation of the infected persons.

The bill sought to:
1. appoint designated health authorities to carryout the provisions of the Act. They can demand information from infected persons and will provide health education, counseling, treatment, social support and rehabilitation;
2. require registered medical practitioners to report cases of HIV infection, drug addicts and AIDS; and
3. provide for the establishment of surveillance centers.

The bill produced many ethical and legal problems and was withdrawn.

Ethical Issues

There are a large number of ethical problems related to AIDS. Some of them are related to HIV testing. There are many others.

1. *When a 'healthy, would-be donor is tested positive for HIV, should the person be told of the result ?*

The donor has the right to choose whether to be told or not. Yet, there is need for him/her to be aware, so as to prevent him or her from infecting others. Would informing a person that he/she tested positive for HIV ensure that the spread of infection will be prevented? This is very doubtful. It is very difficult to change the sexual behavior of a person. So also, it is difficult to stop a professional donor from selling blood at another commercial blood bank.

Once told, the infected individual has to endure all the negative consequences of knowing that he/she is infected. The news will create psychological upheaval in the person. It can result in social ostracisation and discrimination. Will the individual get the benefits, such as psychosocial assistance, prevention and treatment of opportunistic infections and antiviral treatment (however limited the usefulness may be)?

2. *If the person is clinically suspected to be suffering from AIDS, should HIV testing be done?*

If the result of HIV testing will help in deciding on the best course of medical care for the benefit of the person, then the testing should be carried out with counseling.

3. *Can testing be done without informed consent?*

Testing should ordinarily be done only with informed consent. Without informed consent, proper counseling (pre-and post-test) cannot be provided.

In epidemiological surveys, informed consent of the individuals being tested may not be obtained. In such cases, anonymity of the persons screened must be maintained. Their names must not be linked to the results.

4. *Should a doctor reveal the patient's infection to his or her spouse, to his or her children and others living with the patient?*

Giving the information without the consent of the person violates confidentiality. At the same time, it is necessary to protect others and prevent the spread of infection. It has to be done judiciously and with sensitivity. Sudden disclosure can bring on disaster, including suicide and disruption of the family.

If a doctor finds that one of his/her patients is HIV positive but continues to have sexual intercourse with the sexual partner, should the doctor inform the partner of the HIV status? Would it be violation of confidentiality? If the doctor does not inform, will he/she be responsible for exposing the partner to the risk of contracting a fatal infection? If the partner gets infected, can he/she sue the person who infected and the doctor, who knew but did not inform?

In some of the states in USA, it is a crime for an HIV positive person to have sex with a partner without informing the partner of the infection. A similar law exists in Australia.

5. *Can a doctor refuse to treat an AIDS patient or one who is HIV infected ?*

The Medical Council of India Code of Medical Ethics says: "The doctor is not bound to treat each and everyone seeking his services, except in emergencies. He is free to choose whom he will serve". The General Medical Council (UK) says: "It is unethical for a doctor to refuse to treat or examine a patient for the sole reason that the patient's condition may put the doctor at personal risk".

The opinion in USA is: "It is unethical not to give a sick or dying patient appropriate treatment whatever the reason ".

The general consensus is that it is the duty of the doctor to provide all needed medical care to a patient with AIDS, observing all necessary precautions.

6. *How do we allocate resources ?*

We need to allocate resources to prevent spread of infection and to fight the disease, knowing that there is no effective vaccine or medicine at present. Whatever medicine is now available is highly expensive. We also know that the same resources could save the lives of many suffering from the other diseases. A judicious decision must be made.

7. *Can we set up quarantine arrangements for patients with HIV infection ?*

Unlike other infectious diseases, quarantine in the case of patients with HIV infection has to be lifelong. It will be expensive with respect to resources. The prospect of being incarcerated for life could make the patients dodge detection and conceal symptoms. Quarantine (for life) curtails the individual's liberty, guaranteed by the Constitution.

CHAPTER 20 Genetics

We are in a new era of challenges. The human genome has been determind. The newer advances in the science and technology of genetics can help us to counter the outcome of certain genetic defects.

GENETIC TECHNOLOGY

Defects in the genes can produce defects or deficiencies in the gene products leading to diseases or disorders. "Diseases are a consequence of the interaction of the genes with the environment."—Paul Berg, Nobel Laureate.

Genetic technology is used for detecting abnormalities in the fetus, newborn and infant. Sickle cell anemia and thalassemia can be detected early and steps taken. Counseling of couples and parents can reduce genetic abnormalities. Dietary management is possible in some abnormalities. Gene replacement is possible to effect cure.

It is also possible to block the activities of certain genes and thus reduce the production of substances when it is in excess. So also, it is possible to stimulate greater production of deficient substances. But we have to be careful.

Prenatal Diagnosis

There are a number of prenatal diagnostic techniques for detecting genetic or metabolic disorders, chromosomal abnormalities, congenital malformations or sex-linked disorders. These procedures are controlled by the Prenatal Diagnostic Techniques (Regulation and Prevention of Misuse) Act, 1994.

Genetic Counseling Centers/Laboratories/Clinics

These centres/laboratories/clinics must be registered to conduct prenatal diagnostic tests, counseling, etc. The requirements for registration under the Act are set out in the Rules. They should employ only persons with prescribed qualifications and should maintain proper records.

The tests can be conducted, if the pregnant woman:

- is above 35 years of age;
- had two or more spontaneous abortions or fetal loss;
- has been exposed to potentially teratogenic agents (drugs, radiation, infection or chemicals); or
- has a family history of mental retardation or physical deformities, such as spasticity or any other genetic disease.

Consent of Pregnant Woman

The prenatal diagnostic procedures may be conducted only after all known side and after effects of the procedures have been explained to the pregnant woman concerned and her written, free and informed consent to undergo such procedures is obtained in the language understood by her.

Prohibition of Communicating the Sex of the Fetus

The genetic counselling centre/laboratory/clinic or person shall not conduct or cause to be conducted prenatal diagnostic techniques for determining the sex of the fetus. Further, no person conducting prenatal diagnostic procedures shall communicate to the pregnant woman concerned or her relatives, the sex of the fetus by words, signs or in any other manner. Advertisements, in any form relating to prenatal determination of sex is prohibited.

Ethical Issues

A number of ethical issues are involved.

- Proper, regulated conduct of the diagnostic procedures with competence.
- Maintenance of all records.
- Need for free, informed consent for the procedures.
- Prevention of sex determination, discrimination and selective abortion of the female fetus.

Potential candidates for future gene therapy are the disorders caused by defects in a single cell. The cells are removed from the person, the healthy gene is inserted and the cells returned to the body. In *augmentation therapy*, a healthy gene is added. It helps in replacing the product of a missing or defective gene but does not physically replace the faulty DNA. Augmentation is beneficial when a genetic derangement results in little or no production of a product.

Ethical Issues in Use of Genetic Technology

1. Has the individual the right to decide what may be done to his genes or his children's genes to prevent or treat diseases?
2. Does the individual have the right to know his genetic abnormalities, which are not apparent now but may become evident in diseases many years later?
3. If the young woman asks the advice of the specialist about the young man she intends to marry and the young man has a genetic defect which may shorten his life or affect their children, can the specialist divulge the information? Has the specialist the right to refuse to give the information?
4. Can the employer ask for the genome map of the employee or prospective employee, and discharge the employee, if found to have genes which give possible behavioral characteristics, which, according to the employer are not desirable or refuse to give the job based on the genome map?
5. Has the individual the right to refuse to have his or her genome revealed?
6. Is it ethical to obtain the genome map without the informed consent of the individual?

All of these questions and many others will have to be decided using the principles of medical ethics.

As regards germ cells, the ethical decision is that there could be no manipulation of the germ cells involved in reproduction. It will involve interference with genetic inheritance of future generations.

EUGENICS

Eugenics means "well-born". There is often a desire to improve human heredity by:

- selecting and increasing the beneficial qualities, and
- removing or reducing harmful ones.

The dream will be to create a substantial measure of the human person to produce a "superman", possessing extra-ordinary qualities, extraordinary physical powers, extra-sensory perceptions and extraintellectual capabilities. Can biocyborgs be created? Is it desirable to create them?

Eugenics can be positive or negative.

Positive eugenics deals with the development of a new person, through the selection of genotypes from persons possessing exceptional physical and mental qualities. We usually think of persons physically stronger or with strong mental powers and creativity. We seldom think of social and spiritual qualities.

Negative eugenics deals with the study of inheritable diseases and deficiencies. Most of the modern medical eugenics deal with negative eugenics. By genetic engineering and counseling of couples, we try to reduce the likelihood of the development of such diseases as diabetes mellitus.

Positive eugenics makes use of a selection process of gifted persons for improving the human gene pool. It needs control over human reproduction. The right to procreate is determined by others (the State). Gifted persons with "desirable" qualities are allowed and encouraged to procreate; others are not allowed.

Who will decide?

- Who shall be the elite group who can procreate?
- Who shall be denied the right to reproduce?

It is an awful responsibility. It can be abused easily. Often the idea is to have such "outstanding" persons contribute to a sperm bank. Artificial insemination is done with ovum selected from women with "desirable" qualities.

What qualities are desirable? What characteristics are truly worthy in the human? Who will judge? How will society make the choice?

A genetically poor or mediocre but politically powerful dictator may decide to disseminate his genes and then have clones produced. If the individual is sacred and there is inviolability and uniqueness of the human person, then positive eugenics is unethical.

The objective of eugenics is to produce an ideal person. But who is an ideal person? Physical, mental, social and spiritual qualities must be considered. At present, we do not have the knowledge to decide what all will contribute to the making of the ideal person. It is unethical to genetically attempt to 'modify' the human person.

- Our knowledge of genetics is limited.
- Manipulation with nature might bring on genetic catastrophe for the human race.
- Human characteristics depend on genetic and environmental factors. Reliance only on genetic factors can be disastrous.
- Positive eugenics is often resorted to by people (and countries, e.g. Nazi Germany) with racist ideologies.
- Positive eugenics produces distorted views of human being's value. Emphasis is placed on the physical and intellectual qualities leaving out the social and spiritual aspects.

Some people think that, with the unravelling of the human genome, they can select the offspring they want.

"The idea that we will be able to select genes that we like and weed out those we don't to produce customised children is absurd".

—Neil Holtzman, BMJ, 322:1017, 2001

UNIVERSAL DECLARATION ON THE HUMAN GENOME AND HUMAN RIGHTS, 1997

A. HUMAN DIGNITY AND THE HUMAN GENOME

Article 1

The human genome underlies the fundamental unity of all members of the human family, as well as the recognition of their inherent dignity and diversity. In a symbolic sense, it is the heritage of humanity.

Article 2

a. Everyone has a right to respect for their dignity and for their rights regardless of their genetic characteristics.
b. That dignity makes it imperative not to reduce individuals to their genetic characteristics and to respect their uniqueness and diversity.

Article 3

The human genome, which by its nature evolves, is subject to mutations. It contains potentialities that are expressed differently according to each individual's natural and social environment including the individual's state of health, living conditions, nutrition and education.

Article 4

The human genome in its natural state shall not give rise to financial gains.

B. RIGHTS OF THE PERSONS CONCERNED

Article 5

a. Research, treatment or diagnosis affecting an individual's genome shall be undertaken only after rigorous and prior assessment of the potential risks and benefits pertaining thereto and in accordance with any other requirement of national law.

b. In all cases, the prior, free and informed consent of the person concerned shall be obtained. If the latter is not in a position to consent, consent or authorization shall be obtained in the manner prescribed by law, guided by the person's best interest.
c. The right of each individual to decide whether or not to be informed of the results of genetic examination and the resulting consequences should be respected.
d. In the case of research, protocols shall, in addition, be submitted for prior review in accordance with relevant national and international research standards or guidelines.
e. If according to the law a person does not have the capacity to consent, research affecting his or her genome may only be carried out for his or her direct health benefit, subject to the authorization and the protective conditions prescribed by law. Research which does not have an expected direct health benefit may only be undertaken by way of exception, with the utmost restraint, exposing the person only to a minimal risk and minimal burden and if the research is intended to contribute to the health benefit of other persons in the same age category or with the same genetic condition, subject to the conditions prescribed by law, and provided such research is compatible with the protection of the individual's human rights.

Article 6

No one shall be subjected to discrimination based on genetic characteristics that is intended to infringe or has the effect of infringing human rights, fundamental freedoms and human dignity.

Article 7

Genetic data associated with an identifiable person and stored or processed for the purposes of research or any other purpose must be held confidential in the conditions set by law.

Article 8

Every individual shall have the right, according to international and national law, to just reparation for any damage sustained as a direct and determining result of an intervention affecting his or her genome.

Article 9

In order to protect human rights and fundamental freedoms, limitations to the principles of consent and confidentiality may only be prescribed by law, for compelling reasons within the bounds of public international law and the international law of human rights.

C. RESEARCH ON THE HUMAN GENOME

Article 10

No research or research applications concerning the human genome, in particular in the fields of biology, genetics and medicine, should prevail over respect for the human rights, fundamental freedoms and human dignity of individuals or, where applicable, of groups of people.

Article 11

Practices which are contrary to human dignity, such as reproductive cloning of human beings, shall not be permitted. States and competent international organizations are invited to co-operate in identifying such practices and in taking, at national or international level, the measures necessary to ensure that the principles set out in this Declaration are respected.

Article 12

a. Benefits from advances in biology, genetics and medicine, concerning the human genome, shall be made available to all, with due regard for the dignity and human rights of each individual.
b. Freedom of research, which is necessary for the progress of knowledge, is part of freedom of thought. The applications of research, including applications in biology, genetics and medicine, concerning the human genome, shall seek to offer relief from suffering and improve the health of individuals and human kind as a whole.

D. CONDITIONS FOR THE EXERCISE OF SCIENTIFIC ACTIVITY

Article 13

The responsibilities inherent in the activities of researchers, including meticulousness, caution, intellectual honesty and integrity in carrying out their research as well as in the presentation and utilization of their findings, should be the subject of particular attention in the framework of research on the human genome, because of its ethical and social implications. Public and private science policy-makers also have particular responsibilities in this respect.

Article 14

States should take appropriate measures to foster the intellectual and material conditions favourable to freedom in the conduct of research on the human genome and to consider the ethical, legal, social and economic implications of such research, on the basis of the principles set out in this Declaration.

Article 15

States should take appropriate steps to provide the framework for the free exercise of research on the human genome with due regard for the principles set out in this Declaration, in order to safeguard respect for human rights, fundamental freedoms and human dignity and to protect public health. They should seek to ensure that research results are not used for non-peaceful purposes.

Article 16

States should recognize the value of promoting, at various levels, as appropriate, the establishment of independent, multidisciplinary and pluralist ethics committees to assess the ethical, legal and social issues raised by research on the human genome and its application.

E. SOLIDARITY AND INTERNATIONAL CO-OPERATION

Article 17

States should respect and promote the practice of solidarity towards individuals, families and population groups who are particularly vulnerable to or affected by disease or disability of a genetic character. They should foster, *inter alia*, research on the identification, prevention and treatment of genetically-based and genetically-influenced diseases, in particular rare as well as endemic diseases which affect large numbers of the world's population.

Article 18

States should make every effort, with due and appropriate regard for the principles set out in this Declaration, to continue fostering the international dissemination of scientific knowledge concerning the human genome, human diversity and genetic research and, in that regard, to foster scientific and cultural co-operation, particularly between industrialized and developing countries.

Article 19

a. In the framework of international co-operation with developing countries, States should seek to encourage measures enabling:
    i. assessment of the risks and benefits pertaining to research on the human genome to be carried out and abuse to be prevented;
    ii. the capacity of developing countries to carry out research on human biology and genetics, taking into consideration their specific problems, to be developed and strengthened;
    iii. developing countries to benefit from the achievements of scientific and technological research so that their use in favour of economic and social progress can be to the benefit of all;
    iv. the free exchange of scientific knowledge and information in the areas of biology, genetics and medicine to be promoted.
b. Relevant international organizations should support and promote the initiatives taken by States for the above mentioned purposes.

F. PROMOTION OF THE PRINCIPLES SET OUT IN THE DECLARATION

Article 20

States should take appropriate measures to promote the principles set out in the Declaration, through education and relevant means, *inter alia* through the conduct of research and training in interdisciplinary fields and through the promotion of education in bioethics, at all levels, in particular for those responsible for science policies.

Article 21

States should take appropriate measures to encourage other forms of research, training and information dissemination conducive to raising the awareness of society and all of its members of their responsibilities regarding the fundamental issues relating to the defence of human dignity which may be raised by research in biology, in genetics and in medicine, and its applications. They should also undertake to facilitate on this subject an open international discussion, ensuring the free expression of various socio-cultural, religious and philosophical opinions.

G. IMPLEMENTATION OF THE DECLARATION

Article 22

States should make every effort to promote the principles set out in this Declaration and should, by means of all appropriate measures, promote their implementation.

Article 23

States should take appropriate measures to promote, through education, training and information dissemination, respect for the above mentioned principles and to foster their recognition and effective application. States should also encourage exchanges and networks among independent ethics committees, as they are established, to foster full collaboration.

Article 24

The International Bioethics Committee of UNESCO should contribute to the dissemination of the principles set out in this Declaration and to the further examination of issues raised by their applications and by the evolution of the technologies in question. It should organize appropriate consultations with parties concerned, such as vulnerable groups. It should make recommendations, in accordance with UNESCO's statutory procedures, addressed to the General Conference and give advice concerning the follow-up of this Declaration, in particular regarding the identification of practices that could be contrary to human dignity, such as germline interventions.

Article 25

Nothing in this Declaration may be interpreted as implying for any State, group or person any claim to engage in any activity or to perform any act contrary to human rights and fundamental freedoms, including the principles set out in this Declaration.

CHAPTER 21 Human Experimentation

There is need for continuing research, if medical science is to progress. The term research in medicine covers a wide spectrum of activities ranging from a review of case-notes to basic investigations aimed at advancing fundamental knowledge. Research brings benefits to patients (present and future), to the researcher doing the work and to the society. Research may be carried out in the laboratory, on chemicals and equipment, on animals or on humans.

Experiments and trials on human beings are necessary. The results of the laboratory and on animals cannot be applied directly to human beings. Can human experiments be carried out without limitation? How to decide what is right and what is wrong in human experimentation?

HUMAN EXPERIMENTATION

Biomedical research involving human beings is necessary for:
- elucidation of physiological or pathological process in health and disease,
- ascertaining the response to particular intervention, whether drugs and pharmaceuticals cooperative procedures or any other, in an individual, healthy or ill, or
- determining the effect of preventive and therapeutic measures in communities.

We must distinguish between human experimentation, clinical trials and innovative treatment. There are very strict rules regarding human experimentation. The rules are less stringent regarding new treatment likely to bring greater benefits to the patient and when other accepted procedures have not succeeded.

Human experimentation is carried out with many objectives:

- Benefit to the individual human subject involved in the experiment.
- Potential benefit to a group of patients suffering from that disease.
- Long-term benefit to humanity in general.
- Contribution to human knowledge.

In the first instance, the individual benefits. It should be carried out only if experiments in the laboratory and on animals indicate possible beneficial effects. The doctor has to consider the benefits and risks involved. The patient must be considered as a partner in research and not merely as a subject of research.

Research on human beings is regulated by international and national codes of conduct. The first international declaration was *the Nuremberg Code* (1947). It arose out of the Nuremberg trials of Nazi physicians, who participated in cruel experiments on prisoners, those in concentration camps, the mentally retarded persons and others, during the second world war. These amounted to torture, often ending in death. Among the experiments were exposures to extreme cold, submerging the person under water for long periods and exposure to poisons and toxic substances. In 1964, the World Medical Assembly meeting at Helsinki set up a code of conduct, known as the *Helsinki declaration*. This has been modified by the World Medical Assembly at Tokyo in 1975. The Council for International Organizations of Medical Sciences (1982) along with the World Health Organization has given international guidelines for biomedical research involving human subjects.

Even after the Helsinki Declaration, unethical human experimentation continued. An example of unethical research is the Tuskegee Study of Untreated Syphilis, sponsored by the US Public Health Service, lasting from 1932 to 1974. 412 poor African-American men with untreated syphilis were followed and compared with 204 men free of the disease to determine the natural history of the disease. When the study began, the treatment available was not very good but the research continued even after pencillin became widely available. The ethical violations were multiple:

- subjects were not provided with information; there was no informed consent; they were deliberately deceived;
- they were not given the best known treatment;

- the study continued even after the highly effective treatment became available.

The Indian Council of Medical Research (1980) had given detailed guidelines for the conduct of human experiment and research. These have been modified recently (2000) and new comprehensive guidelines have been given.

Important Requisites

Some important requisites for human experimentation are discussed here.

1. Essentiality

The proposed research must be necessary for the benefit of the people and the advancement of knowledge. The principle of essentiality respects the ethical principle of beneficence.

2. Informed Consent

The research subject (or the guardian or legal proxy) should be fully apprised of the proposed research, including the risk and benefit and the alternate procedures available. The free (voluntary) informed consent should be obtained before the commencement of the research. The research subject has the right to abstain from the research at any time. Due care should be taken at all stages of research to ensure minimization of risk. Where the research involves any community or group of persons, the principle of informed consent and voluntariness applies to the community as a whole and to each individual member.

The principle of autonomy is observed by informed consent. It protects the individual's freedom of choice. The extent of information to be given varies with the situation: Research involving only collection of data from the medical records; emergencies; others of similar nature will not call for rigorous application of 'informed consent'.

3. Confidentiality

The identity and particulars of the subject and the research data should be kept confidential. These may be disclosed only for valid reasons: Legal (court orders) or scientific (therapy) and with the specific consent in writing of the subject participating in the research.

4. Compensation

The research protocol shall include mechanisms for compensation through insurance or other appropriate means to cover all risks and provide for remedial action and after-care. It is the duty of the sponsor to provide adequate compensation for any physical or mental injury. In case of death, the dependents are entitled to material compensation. Immediate recompense and rehabilitative measures should be undertaken, when needed. The participants may be paid for:

- inconvenience,
- time away from work, and
- reimbursement of expenses incurred.

The participants may also receive free medical services. Payments should not be so large as to induce the subjects to participate against their better judgement.

5. Competence

The research should be conducted only by competent and qualified persons and who are aware of and practise ethical research. The research must be conducted with integrity.

6. Accountability, Responsibility and Transparency

All persons involved, directly or indirectly, in the research are responsible and accountable for observing all the ethical principles and guidelines. Such persons include:

- the researcher (s),
- the sponsors and funders,
- the institution where the research is conducted, and
- those who use the results of the research.

There should be no conflict of interest. The research should be conducted in a fair, honest, impartial and transparent manner. The complete records of the research should be retained for reasonable period as considered necessary for postresearch monitoring and evaluation.

Institutions conducting research in collaboration with commercial firms should consider possible conflicts of interest (e.g. researcher being a shareholder of the firm developing a new drug).

7. Risk Minimization

Due care must be exercised at every stage of the research, from its inception, design and conduct to the use of the results. The research participant should be subjected to minimum risk and should not suffer from irreversible adverse effects.

8. Scientific Committee

The research proposals must be submitted to a properly constituted scientific committee, who may or may not approve of the proposal, with or without modifications. The scientific committee may review the protocol periodically. Sometimes the functions of the scientific and ethics committees may be combined in a single committee.

9 Ethics Committee

A properly constituted ethics committee shall look into all ethical aspects of the proposed research and may or may not approve of the research, with or without modifications. The ethics committee may review the research procedures periodically. Research on human beings should be conducted observing the basic ethical principles of beneficence, non-maleficence, justice and autonomy.

10. Institutional Arrangements

The institutions involved shall make all necessary arrangements for the proper conduct of research and storage and use of the data and for ensuring confidentiality.

11. Publication of Results

The results of research (positive or negative) should be available to the public through scientific or other publications. The information given should be accurate. It should not raise false hopes or expectations. Confidentiality must be maintained while publishing/presenting the results.

12. Special Groups as Research Subjects

Pregnant and nursing women should not be subjects of any clinical trial except when such trials are designed to protect or promote their health and for which non-pregnant or non-nursing women are not suitable.

Children will not be involved in research that could be carried out equally well with adults. Children will be involved if the purpose of the research is to obtain specific information relevant to the health needs of children and, in the case of drug trials, the drug has therapeutic value in a primary disease of children.

Vulnerable groups with reduced autonomy, such as students, employees, service personnel and prisoners, may be involved in research, only if there is adequate justification. Their vulnerability should not be exploited.

Rights and welfare of the mentally ill or the mentally retarded should be protected at all times.

Persons who are economically or socially disadvantaged should not be used to benefit those who are better off than such persons.

Community Based Research

In research involving the whole or a major part of the community, it will not be possible to get the informed consent of everyone. This often involves public health measures. The public health authority has the final responsibility which should not be taken lightly. Ethical considerations require that all aspects including the likely benefits and risks of the proposed research are considered carefully.

The research is undertaken only after informing the community affected and obtaining their general consent through the leaders, elected representatives and other individuals.

Examples of community based research are:

- experimental treatment of drinking water (e.g. fluorides),
- large scale experimental immunization with new vaccines (e.g. vaccines against leprosy),
- nutritional supplements (e.g. iodized salt), and
- vector control (e.g. filariasis).

All the above produce controversies,whether it be fluoridization of drinking water, iodisation of salt or vaccine trials. The controversies may be with respect to the need or advisability because of other sideeffects. It could also be in the methodology. There may also be social reasons.

A large scale trial of three different vaccines against leprosy was to be conducted in one of the districts (endemic for leprosy) in Tamil Nadu. Two of the vaccines have been developed in

India (the ICRC and MW vaccines) and the third one is the WHO sponsored BCG plus killed *M. leprae* vaccine. The tests were to be carried out on 250,000 people in 150 villages, excluding infants below 1 year, pregnant women and those above 65 years. The inclusion of the WHO sponsored vaccine created a controversy. This vaccine was under trial in Venezuela. Why try it here before the results of that trial were known? Many felt that it was being included under pressure from WHO and not for valid scientific reasons.

The community may sometimes identify certain problems of health which are important from their view point. It must be possible to carry out research on such problems. Community participation can be expected to be high in such instances.

Ethical review committee: Constitute an ethical review committee. There can be national, local or institutional review committees.

The committee must have appropriate representation: Medical and non-medical. The committee should have the authority to take independent decisions.

The research proposal must be scientifically sound. If it is not, it is unethical to use it. If scientifically sound, ethical soundness must be considered. This is done by the ethical review committee. The committee must consider all ethical aspects of the proposed research.

Ethical review committee must be specially strict in the case of children, pregnant and nursing mothers, mentally defective or ill and subjects who cannot refuse easily, or are not familiar with the implications of biomedical research.

Researches Sponsored by Outside Agencies

Clinical trials are becoming big business in India. For a variety of reasons such trials are being transferred by Transnational Corporations to India. It is necessary to ensure that such studies do not compromise on the scientific and ethical principles.

The Department of Health and Human Services Regulations governing US sponsored research in foreign countries and the Joint Guidelines for Research in the Third World issued by WHO and the Council for International Organizations of Medical Sciences state: Human subjects should receive protection atleast equivalent to that in the sponsoring country.

Many studies are carried out in the Third World that could not be done in the countries sponsoring the work. A group of patients at the Regional Cancer Centre, Thiruvananthapuram had been subjected to trials with a drug, M N developed at the John's Hopkins University, USA, even though the Federal Drugs Administration, USA, had removed it from "Generally regarded as safe" category. Such trials were not being carried out in USA. The study had been carried out at the center for 2 years, till one of the doctors at the center petitioned the State Human Rights Commission. The John's Hopkins University, on becoming aware of the situation, said that the faculty member had been directed to cease all activities related to the study and that the University had not approved the study. The University ordered an enquiry. The preliminary enquiry found that the study had not been authorized by any department of the University; "it had not been reviewed or approved by any of the University's institutional review boards concerned with the protection of human subjects". -—Indian Express, Mumbai, 31 July, 2001.

When researches are sponsored, financed and conducted fully or partially by outside agencies in collaboration with researchers in the host country, ensure that:

- the ethical norms of the initiating (sponsoring) and host countries are fully met, and
- the protocol submitted by the researchers of the initiating country is approved by the ethical review committees in the initiating country and the host country.

Review Procedures

There must be constant review of the effects of the experiment. Safety must be assessed constantly.

Compensation for Accidental Injury

Though rare, should accidents occur, the participant must be compensated quickly and adequately. Experimental subjects should not be asked to waive their rights to compensation, when giving their willingness to participate.

Protocol

When submitting the protocol, the investigators must provide complete and correct information.

- Objectives of the research together with the state of knowledge, what gap is expected to be filled and the justification for carrying out the investigation.
- Evidence that the investigators are adequately qualified and experienced.
- Design of the experiment including the number and type of participants and duration of the experiment.
- Criteria for inclusion of experimental subject including the procedure for obtaining free informed consent.
- Relevant laboratory and animal experiments carried out with the drug or procedure.
- Probable benefits and risks to the participants.
- Maintenance of confidentiality.
- Declaration that all ethical principles will be followed.

Institutional Ethics Committee/Institutional Review Board

All proposals on biomedical research involving human beings should be cleared by the Institutional Ethics Committee. The main objective of the Committee is to safeguard the welfare and rights of the participants in the research. It is advisable to have a Scientific Reveiw Committee, which will consider the scientific aspects of the proposed research. Once the proposal is approved from the scientific angle, the proposal is placed before the Ethics Committee.

Responsibilities

The Ethics Committee is responsible to:

- protect the rights, safety and well-being of the potential research participants,
- obtain the following documents:
  - trial protocols, updated with amendments, if any
  - written informed consent
  - subject recruitment procedures
  - written information to be provided to the subjects
  - safety information
  - compensation available, if mishaps occur and
  - curriculum vitae of the investigators.
- ensure that the ethical principles are applied in relation to the local values and customs;

- provide consultation to the professional staff and patients/families on ethical issues and problems;
- provide education and advice to the staff, patients/families;
- initiate and, on request, formulate policies on the ethical aspects of clinical care at organisational level;
- conduct seminars/workshops periodically for all categories of hospital personnel regarding ethical concerns.

Hospital Ethics Committee

The Hospital Ethics Committee is responsible to ensure that the hospital provides the best possible medical care.

- Bedside care
- Relief of suffering
- Cure of disease
- Prevention of iatrogenic disease
- Cost to patient: Tests, drugs, other costs; avoiding unnecessary expenditure
- Attention to the needs of the patient
- Care of seriously ill
- Dying and dead patient
- Education of the staff; seminars/workshops on ethics
- Brain death
- Harvesting organs for transplantation
- Informed consent
- Forum for redressal of complaints; ombudsman
- Patient's rights
- Citizen's rights
- Standards of care

Functions of Hospital Ethics Committee: They relate to:

- Patient care
- Research
- Education of faculty and other personnel.

Education

The aim is to provide the hospital staff with the concepts, principles and body of knowledge about ethics to enable them to address the complex ethical dimensions of hospital practice: provider: patient relationship; ethical rights of patients and their families; ethical obligations of the providers to the profession/patients/families/society. The committee assists the hospital in the development of policies and guidelines regarding recurrent ethical issues, questions or problems which arise in the care of patients.

Case Review

The Committee can set as a forum for analysis of ethical questions which arise in the care of individual patients. The committee provides support to those responsible for treatment decisions—healthcare providers, patients, surrogates and members of the patient's family. The decisions may involve:

- those of ethical ambiguity;
- disagreement between care providers or between providers and patients/families regarding the ethical aspects of patient care; or
- withholding or withdrawal of life-sustaining treatment.

Educational Functions

Own education: Provide members information about clinical ethics and access to the rapidly expanding literature in this field.

- Orientation of new members
- Specific reading assignments
- Seminars
- Hospital community

Composition: It has to be multidisciplinary. The more diverse the members, the more enriching will be their viewpoints.

- Clinicians
- Basic scientists
- Social worker
- Nurse
- Rehabilitation personnel
- Priest/philosopher/ethicist
- Lawyer/retired judge
- Administration
- A respected member of the public who has no professional or institutional ties with the hospital.

CHAPTER 22

Clinical Trials

Evaluation of drugs is done after studying the new drugs in the laboratory and in animals. Clinical trials of drugs/vaccines are designed to evaluate the effectiveness and safety of drugs/vaccines, the dosage, route of administration, etc. All drug trials will be conducted in accordance with the guidelines of the Indian Council of Medical Research and the International Conference on Harmonization Guidelines for Good Clinical Practice (1996). The trial should be carried out only after receiving the approval of the Drugs Controller General of India. It is also necessary to get the approval of the Ethics Committee of the Institution. There is need for separate clinical trials in the country before the drug is approved for marketing, even if trials had been carried out in the country where the drug had been developed. There can be variations in metabolism, responses and toxicity.

Phases of Clinical Trials of Drugs

1. Phase I is done in volunteers to determine the safety of the maximum tolerated dose in healthy adults. At least two subjects are given each dose to establish.
   - the safe dosage range,
   - pharmacokinetic and pharmacodynamic effects, and
   - adverse drug reactions, if any.
2. Phase II trials are controlled studies conducted in a limited number of patients to determine therapeutic uses, effective dose range and further evaluation of safety and pharmacokinetics. 20–25 patients are studied for assessment of each dosage.
3. Phase III trials have the objective of obtaining enough data about the efficacy and safety of drugs in a large number of

patients, usually in comparison with a standard drug. If a standard drug is not available, it is done in comparison with a placebo. If Phase III trials are successful, permission may be granted for marketing the drug.

4. After approval for marketing, postmarketing surveillance (phase IV) is undertaken to obtain additional information about the drug's risks and benefits. Adverse reactions, if any, should be brought to the notice of the Ethics Committee.

Clinical Trials of Vaccines

1. Phase I involves the introduction of the vaccine into the human population for determination of its safety and biological effects including immunogenecity. It includes the study of the dose and route of administration.
2. Phase II involves the study of the effectiveness (immunogenecity) in a limited number of volunteers. Prophylactic vaccines are given to normal volunteers; therapeutic or curative vaccines are given to patients suffering from the disease.
3. Phase III focuses on assessment of safety and effectiveness in the prevention of disease. It involved controlled study on a very large number of volunteers.

Some Special Concerns

- Vaccines that contain active or live-attenuated micro-organisms may produce infection. The subject to be vaccinated should be informed of the same.
- The subjects in the control groups run the risk of contracting the disease.

The Investigator

The Investigator(s) should be competent in conducting the trial properly (qualification, training and experience). He/she should be thoroughly familiar with the investigational product, as described in the protocol, product information and other information provided by the sponsor, as also the regulatory requirements. The investigator should have the needed resources and ensure that all persons assisting with the trial have the necessary information about the duties and functions related to the trial.

The investigator/institution should ensure good medical care of the subject, especially for any adverse reactions.

If a subject withdraws from the investigation, the investigator should try to ascertain the reason, while fully respecting the right of the subject not to give any reason.

The investigator should maintain complete records of the investigational product which should be stored as specified by the sponsor and used only in accordance with the approved protocol.

The investigator should ensure the accuracy and completeness of all the data collected, and should maintain the trial documents, as required.

Informed Consent

No undue influence should be brought on the subject to participate in the trial. The consent form should not contain any word/ phrase/sentence which would appear to waive the rights of the subject or release the investigator, institution or sponsor from liability for negligence. The investigator or a responsible person designated by the investigator should fully inform the subject of all relevant aspects of the trial. The language used in the consent form should be as non-technical as feasible and in a form and language easily understood by the subject. The subject should be amply provided with opportunity to ask questions about the trial and get satisfactory answers. The written informed consent form should be signed and dated by the subject personally prior to participation in the trial (if the subject is unable to read and write, an impartial witness should be present throughout the entire informed consent discussion. The informed consent form and related documents should be read and explained to the subject, in a language understood by the subject. The witness should sign and personally date the consent form. The witness attests that the information was adequately explained to the subject and that it was apparently understood by the subject and the informed consent was given freely). The informed consent discussion should include explanations on the following:

- the subject's participation in the trial is purely voluntary and he/she may withdraw at any time, without penalty or loss of benefits

- the records identifying the subject will be kept confidential but the persons involved in the trial will have access to the records without violating the confidentiality of the subject
- the person to contact for further information and in the event of trial-related injury
- the expected duration of the trial and when the subject must be available for the trial
- the trial involves research and experimentation
- the purpose of the trial
- the trial treatment:
  - the probability of random assignment
  - the procedures
  - subject's responsibilities
  - foreseeable risks/inconveniences/benefits
- alternative treatments/procedures and their potential benefits/risks
- compensation and/or treatment available to the subject in the event of trial related injury.

(In instances where the subject is incompetent to consent, due to age, mental deficiency or any other reason, the subject's legally acceptable representative must be involved fully).

Human Embryos

There are increasing reports of experimentation on the human embryos, whether in vivo or in vitro. With in vitro fertilization, when many ova are fertilised at a time and only a few are used for implantation, many embryos become available. Keeping alive the embryo merely for experimental purposes and carrying out experiments not for the benefit of the developing individual are opposed to human dignity and respect for life.

Sometimes, the developing embryo in the uterus may have developmental defects. If the motive for experimentation on the human fetus is for therapeutic purposes bringing benefit to the individual, the procedure is ethically sound. Care should be exercised to ensure that the expected benefit to the individual justified taking the risks involved in the procedure.

The Warnock committee (UK) stated that an embryo is a potential person and that there is a widely shared sentiment that embryo experiments are wrong. They wanted embryo research to be controlled whether financed from public or private funds. No research was to be done on embryos more than 12 days old. No embryo which had been experimented upon should be returned to a woman.

Fraudulent Research

Unfortunately there is considerable amount of fraudulent research going on throughout the world. Cheating in medical research is not uncommon anywhere in the world. There is fabrication of data, plagiarism of articles and inventions as also manipulation and suppression of facts. How can we investigate it? How can we prevent such dishonest practices? One step would be to teach students research ethics. The need for integrity in research cannot be overemphasised. The ethics committees may look into all instances of alleged bogus research. Each institution, where research is carried on, may appoint a person of high standing to receive allegations and screen them. If there is a prima facie case, a three member committee may be appointed to investigate the allegation. There is need to maintain confidentiality and see that natural justice is not violated.

DECLARATION OF HELSINKI

Recommendations guiding medical doctors in biomedical research involving human subjects

Adopted by the 18th World Medical Assembly, Helsinki, Finland, 1964 and as revised by the 29th World Medical Assembly, Tokyo, 1975, Venice, 1983 and Hong Kong, 1989.

Introduction

It is the mission of the medical doctor to safeguard the health of the people. His or her knowledge and conscience are dedicated to the fulfilment of this mission.

The Declaration of Geneva of the World Medical Association binds the doctor with the words, "The health of my patients will be my first consideration", and the International Code of Medical Ethics declares that, "Any art or advice which could weaken physical or mental resistance of a human being may be used only in his interest".

The purpose of biomedical research involving human subjects must be to improve diagnostic, therapeutic and prophylactic procedures and the understanding of the etiology and pathogenesis of disease.

In current medical practice, most diagnostic, therapeutic or prophylactic procedures involve hazards. This applies *a fortiori to* biomedical research.

Medical progress is based on research which ultimately must rest in part on experimentation involving human subjects.

In the field of biomedical research, a fundamental distinction must be recognized between medical research in which the aim is essentially diagnostic or therapeutic for a patient, and medical research, the essential object of which is purely scientific and without direct diagnostic or therapeutic value to the person subjected to the research.

Special caution must be exercised in the conduct of research which may affect the environment, and the welfare of animals used for research must be respected.

Because it is essential that the results of laboratory experiments be applied to human beings to further scientific knowledge and to help suffering humanity, the World Medical Association has prepared the following recommendations as a guide to every doctor in biomedical research involving human subjects. They should be kept under review in the future. It must be stressed that the standards as drafted are only a guide to physicians all over the world. Doctors are not relieved from criminal, civil and ethical responsibilities under the laws of their own countries.

Basic Principles

1. Biomedical research involving human subjects must conform to generally accepted scientific principles and should be based on adequately performed laboratory and animal experimentation and on a thorough knowledge of the scientific literature.
2. The design and performance of each experimental procedure involving human subjects should be clearly formulated in an experimental protocol which should be transmitted to a specially appointed independent committee for consideration, comment and guidance.

3. Biomedical research involving human subjects should be conducted only by scientifically qualified persons and under the supervision of a clinically competent medical person. The responsibility for the human subject must always rest with a medically qualified person and never rest on the subject of the research, even though the subject has given his or her consent.
4. Biomedical research involving human subjects cannot legitimately be carried out unless the importance of the objective is in proportion to the 'inherent risk of the subject.
5. Every biomedical research project involving human subjects should be preceded by careful assessment of predictable risks in comparison with foreseeable benefits to the subjects or to others. Concern for the interests of the subjects must always prevail over the interest of science and society.
6. The right of the research subject to safeguard his or her integrity must always be respected. Every precaution should be taken to respect the privacy of the subject and to minimize the impact of the study on the subject's physical and mental integrity and on the personality of the subject.
7. Doctors should abstain from engaging in research projects involving human subjects unless they are satisfied that the hazards involved are believed to be predictable. Doctors should cease any investigation if the hazards are found to outweigh the potential benefits.
8. In publication of the results of his or her research, the doctor is obliged to preserve the accuracy of the result. Reports of experimentation not in accordance with the principles laid down in this Declaration should not be accepted for publication.
9. In any research on human beings, each potential subject must be adequately informed of the aims, methods, anticipated benefits and potential hazards of the study and the discomfort it may entail. He or she should be informed that he or she is at liberty to abstain from participation in the study and that he or she is free to withdraw his or her consent to participation at any time. The doctor should then obtain the subject's freely given informed consent, preferably in writing.
10. When obtaining informed consent for the research project the doctor should be particularly cautious if the subject is in a

dependent relationship to him or her or may consent under duress. In that case, the informed consent should be obtained by a doctor who is not engaged in the investigation and who is completely independent of this official relationship.

11. In case of legal incompetence, informed consent should be obtained from the legal guardian in accordance with national legislation. Where physical or mental incapacity makes it impossible to obtain informed consent, or when the subject is a minor, permission from the responsible relative replaces that of the subject in accordance with national legislation.
12. The research protocol should always contain a statement of the ethical considerations involved and should indicate that the principles enunciated in the present Declaration are complied with.

Use of Placebo

Many clinical trials were being conducted comparing the benefits of the therapy under trial against placebo administered to the subjects in the control group. The World Medical Association (WMA) became concerned about the use of placebo as control and declared in Helsinki Declaration's paragraph 29 that new treatments should be tested against the best available treatment and not a placebo, unless no proven treatment exists. This was to ensure that the control subjects are not denied the benefits of available therapy. But it created a controversy and WMA issued a clarification:

Clarification of Paragraph 29 of the WMA Declaration of Helsinki (WMA Council, 7 October, 2001, France)

"The WMA is concerned that paragraph 29 of the revised Declaration of Helsinki (Oct, 2000) has led to diverse interpretations and possible confusion. It hereby reaffirms its position that extreme care must be taken in making use of a placebo-controlled trial and that in general, this methodology should only be used in the absence of existing proven therapy. However, a placebo-controlled trial may be ethically acceptable, even if proven therapy is available, under the following circumstances:

- where for compelling and scientifically sound methodological reasons its use is necessary to determine the efficacy or safety of a prophylactic, diagnostic or therapeutic method; or

- where a prophylactic, diagnostic or therapeutic method is being investigated for a minor condition and the patients who receive placebo will not be subject to any additional risk of serious or irreversible harm.

All other provisions of the Declaration of Helsinki must be adhered to, especially the need for appropriate ethical and scientific review".

Medical Research Combined with Professional Care (Clinical Research)

1. In the treatment of the sick person, the doctor must be free to use a new diagnostic and therapeutic measure, if in his or her judgement it offers hope of saving life, reestablishing health or alleviating suffering.
2. The potential benefits, hazards and discomfort of a new method should be weighed against the advantages of the best current diagnostic and therapeutic methods.
3. In any medical study, every patient, including those of a control group if any, should be assured of the best proven diagnostic and therapeutic method.
4. The refusal of the patient to participate in a study must never interfere with the doctor-patient relationship.
5. If the doctor considers it essential not to obtain informed consent, the specific reasons for this proposal should be stated in the experimental protocol for transmission to the independent committee.
6. The doctor can combine medical research with professional care, the objective being the acquisition of new medical knowledge, only to the extent that medical research is justified by its potential diagnostic or therapeutic value for the patient.

NON-THERAPEUTIC BIOMEDICAL RESEARCH

Involving Human Subjects (Non-clinical Biomedical Research)

1. In the purely scientific application of medical research carried out on a human being, it is the duty of the doctor to remain the protector of the life and health of that person on whom biomedical research is being carried out.

2. The subjects should be volunteers either healthy persons or patients for whom the experimental design is not related to the patient's illness.
3. The investigator or the investigating team should discontinue the research if in his/her or their judgement it may, if continued, be harmful to the individual.
4. In research on man, the interest of science and society should never take precedence over considerations related to the well-being of the subject.

Informed consent is an important factor in complying with the guidelines of the Declaration of Helsinki. Often it falls short of the requirements. A study, published in the *British Medical Journal* (1991) showed that there are shortfalls even in countries like Sweden where the awareness is greater among the researchers and the praticipants. The quality of information understood by the participants did not meet the guidelines fully.

Annexure

Indian Medical Council

(Professional Conduct, Etiquettes and Ethics) Requlations, 2002

Ammended up to 8th October, 2018

MEDICAL COUNCIL OF INDIA

NOTIFICATION

New Delhi dated the 11th march, 2002

No. MCI. 211 (2) 2001 – Reg. In exercise of the powers conferred under Section 20A read with Section 33(m) of the Indian Medical Council Act, 1956 (102 of 1956), the Medical Council of India, with the previous approval of the Central Government, hereby makes the following regulations relating to the Professional Conduct, Etiquette and Ethics for registered medical practitioners, namely:

Short Title and Commencement: (1) These regulations may be called the Indian Medical Council (Professional conduct, Etiquette and Ethics) Regulations, 2002.

(2) They shall come into force on the date of their publication in the Official Gazette.

CHAPTER I

1. CODE OF MEDICAL ETHICS

A. Declaration

Each applicant, at the time of making an application for registration under the provisions of the Act, shall be provided a copy of the declaration and shall submit a duly signed Declaration as provided in Appendix 1. The applicant shall also certify that he/she had read and agreed to abide by the same.

B. Duties and Responsibilities of the Physician in General

1.1 Character of Physician (Doctors with qualification of MBBS or MBBS with postgraduate degree/diploma or with equivalent qualification in any medical discipline):

1.1.1 A physician shall uphold the dignity and honor of his profession.

1.1.2 The prime object of the medical profession is to render service to humanity; reward or financial gain is a subordinate consideration. Who-so-ever chooses his profession, assumes the obligation to conduct himself in accordance with its ideals. A physician should be an upright man, instructed in the art of healings. He shall keep himself pure in character and be diligent in caring for the sick; he should be modest, sober, patient, prompt in discharging his duty without anxiety; conducting himself with propriety in his profession and in all the actions of his life.

1.1.3 No person other than a doctor having qualification recognised by Medical Council of India and registered with Medical Council of India/ State Medical Council(s) is allowed to practice Modern System of Medicine or Surgery. A person obtaining qualification in any other System of Medicine is not allowed to practice Modern System of Medicine in any form.

1.2 Maintaining Good Medical Practice

1.2.1 The principal objective of the medical profession is to render service to humanity with full respect for the dignity of profession and man. Physicians should merit the confidence of patients entrusted to their care, rendering to each a full measure of service and devotion. Physicians should try continuously to improve medical knowledge and skills and should make available to their patients and colleagues the benefits of their professional attainments. The physician should practice methods of healing founded on scientific basis and should not associate professionally with any one who violates this principle. The honored ideals of the medical profession imply that the responsibilities of the physician extend not only to individuals but also to society.

1.2.2 Membership in Medical Society: For the advancement of his profession, a physician should affiliate with associations and societies of allopathic medical professions and involve actively in the functioning of such bodies.

1.2.3 A physician should participate in professional meetings as part of Continuing Medical Education Programs, for at least 30 hours every five years, organized by reputed professional academic bodies or any other authorized organizations. The compliance of this requirement shall be informed regularly to Medical Council of India or the State Medical Councils as the case may be.

1.3 Maintenance of Medical Records

1.3.1 Every physician shall maintain the medical records pertaining to his/her indoor patients for a period of 3 years from the date of commencement of the treatment in a standard proforma laid down by the Medical Council of India.

1.3.2 If any request is made for medical records either by the patients/ authorized attendant or legal authorities involved, the same may be duly acknowledged and documents shall be issued within the period of 72 hours.

1.3.3 A registered medical practitioner shall maintain a Register of Medical Certificates giving full details of certificates issued. When issuing a medical certificate he/she shall always enter the identification marks of the patient and keep a copy of the certificate. He/she shall not omit to record the signature and/or thumbmark, address and at least one identification mark of the patient on the medical certificates or report.

1.3.4 Efforts shall be made to computerize medical records for quick retrieval.

1.4 Display of Registration Numbers

1.4.1 Every physician shall display the registration number accorded to him by the State Medical Council/Medical Council of India in his clinic and in all his prescriptions, certificates, money receipts given to his patients.

1.4.2 Physicians shall display as suffix to their names only recognized medical degrees or such certificates/diplomas and memberships/honors which confer professional knowledge or recognizes any exemplary qualification/achievements.

1.5 Use of Generic Names of Drugs: "Every physician should prescribe drugs with generic names legibly and preferably in capital letters and he/she shall ensure that there is a rational prescription and use of drugs".

1.6 Highest Quality Assurance in Patient Care: Every physician should aid in safeguarding the profession against admission to it of those who are deficient in moral character or education. Physician shall not employ in connection with his professional practice any attendant who is neither registered nor enlisted under the Medical Acts in force and shall not permit such persons to attend, treat or perform operations upon patients wherever professional discretion or skill is required.

1.7 Exposure of Unethical Conduct: A physician should expose, without fear or favour, incompetent or corrupt, dishonest or unethical conduct on the part of members of the profession.

1.8 Payment of Professional Services: The physician, engaged in the practice of medicine shall give priority to the interests of patients. The personal financial interests of a physician should not conflict with the medical interests of patients. A physician should announce his fees before rendering service and not after the operation or treatment is under way. Remuneration received for such services should be in the form and amount specifically announced to the patient at the time the service is rendered. It is unethical to enter into a contract of "no cure no payment". Physician rendering service on behalf of the state shall refrain from anticipating or accepting any consideration.

1.9 Evasion of Legal Restrictions: The physician shall observe the laws of the country in regulating the practice of medicine and shall also not assist others to evade such regulations in the interest of public health. A physician should observe the provisions of the State Acts like Drugs and Cosmetics Act, 1940; Pharmacy Act, 1948; Narcotic Drugs and Psychotropic Substances Act, 1985; Medical Termination of Pregnancy Act, 1971; Transplantation of Human Organ Act, 1994; Mental Health Act, 1987; Environmental Protection Act, 1986; Prenatal Sex Determination Techniques Act, 1994; Drugs and Magic Remedies

(Objectionable Advertisement) Act, 1954; Persons with Disabilities Act and Rules, 1998 and such other Acts, Rules, Regulations made by the Central/ State Governments or local Administrative Bodies or any other relevant Act relating to the protection and promotion of public health.

CHAPTER 2

2. DUTIES OF PHYSICIANS TO THEIR PATIENTS

2.1 Obligations to the Sick

2.1.1 Though a physician is not bound to treat each and every person asking his services, he should not only be ever ready to respond to the calls of the sick and the injured, but should be mindful of the high character of his mission and the responsibility he discharges in the course of his professional duties. In his treatment, he should never forget that the health and the lives of those entrusted to his care depend on his skill and attention. A physician should endeavor to add to the comfort of the sick by making his visits at the hour indicated to the patients. A physician advising a patient to seek service of another physician is acceptable; however, in case of emergency a physician must treat the patient. No physician shall arbitrarily refuse treatment to a patient. However, for good reason, when a patient is suffering from an ailment which is not within the range of experience of the treating physician, the physician may refuse treatment and refer the patient to another physician.

2.1.2 Medical practitioner having any incapacity detrimental to the patient or which can affect his performance vis-à-vis the patient is not permitted to practice his profession.

2.2 Patience, Delicacy and Secrecy: Patience and delicacy should characterize the physician. Confidences concerning individual or domestic life entrusted by patients to a physician and defects in the disposition or character of patients observed during medical attendance should never be revealed unless their revelation is required by the laws of the sate. Sometimes, however, a physician must determine whether his duty to society requires him to employ knowledge, obtained through confidence as a physician, to protect a healthy person against a communicable disease to which he is about to be exposed. In such instance, the physician should act as he would wish another to act toward one of his own family in like circumstances.

2.3 Prognosis: The physician should neither exaggerate nor minimize the gravity of a patient's condition. He should ensure himself that the patient, his relatives or his responsible friends have such knowledge of the patient's condition as will serve the best interests of the patient and the family.

2.4 The Patient must not be Neglected: A physician is free to choose whom he will serve. He should, however, respond to any request for his assistance in an emergency. Once having undertaken a case, the physician should not neglect the patient, nor should he withdraw from the case without giving adequate notice to the patient and his family. Provisionally or fully registered medical practitioner shall not willfully commit an act of negligence that may deprive his patient or patients from necessary medical care.

2.5 Engagement for an Obstetric Case: When a physician who has been engaged to attend an obstetric case is absent and another is sent for and delivery accomplished, the acting physician is entitled to his professional fees, but should secure the patient's consent to resign on the arrival of the physician engaged.

CHAPTER 3

3. DUTIES OF PHYSICIAN IN CONSULTATION

3.1 Unnecessary Consultations should be Avoided

3.1.1 However, in case of serious illness and in doubtful or difficult conditions, the physician should request consultation, but under any circumstances such consultation should be justifiable and in the interest of the patient only and not for any other consideration.

3.1.2 Consulting pathologists/radiologists or asking for any other diagnostic laboratory investigation should be done judiciously and not in a routine manner.

3.2 Consultation for Patient's Benefit: In every consultation, the benefit to the patient is of foremost importance. All physicians engaged in the case should be frank with the patient and his attendants.

3.3 Punctuality in Consultation: Utmost punctuality should be observed by a physician in making themselves available for consultations.

3.4 Statement to Patient after Consultation

3.4.1 All statements to the patient or his representatives should take place in the presence of the consulting physicians, except as otherwise agreed. The disclosure of the opinion to the patient or his relatives or friends shall rest with the medical attendant.

3.4.2 Differences of opinion should not be divulged unnecessarily but when there is irreconcilable difference of opinion the circumstances should be frankly and impartially explained to the patient or his relatives or friends. It would be open to them to seek further advice as they so desire.

3.5 Treatment after Consultation: No decision should restrain the attending physician from making such subsequent variations in the treatment if any unexpected change occurs, but at the next consultation, reasons for the variations should be discussed/explained. The same privilege, with its obligations, belongs to the consultant when sent for in an emergency during the absence of attending physician. The attending physician may prescribe medicine at any time for the patient, whereas the consultant may prescribe only in case of emergency or as an expert when called for.

3.6 Patients Referred to Specialists: When a patient is referred to a specialist by the attending physician, a case summary of the patient should be given to the specialist, who should communicate his opinion in writing to the attending physician.

3.7 Fees and other charges

3.7.1 A physician shall clearly display his fees and other charges on the board of his chamber and/or the hospital he is visiting. Prescription should also make clear if the physician himself dispensed any medicine.

3.7.2 A physician shall write his name and designation in full along with registration particulars in his prescription letter head.

Note: In government hospital where the patient-load is heavy, the name of the prescribing doctor must be written below his/her signature.

CHAPTER 4

4. RESPONSIBILITIES OF PHYSICIANS TO EACH OTHER

4.1 Dependence of Physicians on Each Other: A physician should consider it as a pleasure and privilege to render gratuitous service to all physicians and other immediate family dependants.

4.2 Conduct in Consultation: In consultations, no insincerity, rivalry or envy should be indulged in. All due respect should be observed towards the physician in-charge of the case and no statement or remark be made, which would impair the confidence reposed in him. For this purpose no discussion should be carried on in the presence of the patient or his representatives.

4.3 Consultant not to Take Charge of the Case: When a physician has been called for consultation, the consultant should normally not take charge of the case, especially on the solicitation of the patient or friends. The consultant shall not criticize the referring physician. He/she shall discuss the diagnosis/treatment plan with the referring physician.

4.4 Appointment of Substitute: Whenever a physician requests another physician to attend his patients during his temporary absence from his practice, professional courtesy requires the acceptance of such appointment only when he has the capacity to discharge the additional responsibility along with his/her other duties. The physician acting under such an appointment should give the utmost consideration to the interests and reputation of the absent physician and all such patients should be restored to the case of the latter upon his/her return.

4.5 Visiting Another Physician's Case: When it becomes the duty of a physician occupying an official position to see and report upon an illness or injury, he should communicate to the physician in attendance so as to give him an option of being present. The medical officer/physician occupying an official position should avoid remarks upon the diagnosis or the treatment that has been adopted.

CHAPTER 5

5. DUTIES OF PHYSICIAN TO THE PUBLIC AND TO THE PARAMEDICAL PROFESSION

5.1 Physicians as Citizens: Physicians, as good citizens, possessed of special training should disseminate advice on public health issues. They should play their part in enforcing the laws of the community and in sustaining the institutions that advance the interests of humanity. They should particularly cooperate with the authorities in the administration of sanitary/public health laws and regulations.

5.2 Public and Community Health: Physicians, especially those engaged in public health work, should enlighten the public concerning quarantine regulations and measures for the prevention of epidemic and communicable diseases. At all times the physician should notify the constituted public health authorities of every case of communicable disease under his care, in accordance with the laws, rules and regulations of the health authorities. When an epidemic occurs a physician should not abandon his duty for fear of contracting the disease himself.

5.3 Pharmacists/Nurses: Physicians should recognize and promote the practice of different paramedical services such as, pharmacy and nursing as professions and should seek their cooperation wherever required.

CHAPTER 6

6. UNETHICAL ACTS: A physician shall not aid or abet or commit any of the following acts which shall be construed as unethical.

6.1 Advertising

6.1.1 Soliciting of patients directly or indirectly, by a physician, by a group of physicians or by institutions or organizations is unethical. A physician shall not make use of him/her (or his/her name) as subject of any form or manner of advertising or publicity through any mode either alone or in conjunction with others which is of such a character as to invite attention to him or to his professional position, skill, qualification, achievements, attainments, specialities, appointments, associations, affiliations or honors and/or of such character as would ordinarily result in his self aggrandisement. A physician shall not give to any person, whether for compensation or otherwise, any approval, recommendation, endorsement, certificate, report or statement with respect of any drug, medicine, nostrum remedy, surgical, or therapeutic article, apparatus or appliance or any commercial product or article with respect of any property, quality or use thereof or any test, demonstration or trial thereof, for use in connection with his name, signature, or photograph in any form or manner of advertising through any mode nor shall he boast of cases, operations, cures or remedies or permit the publication of report thereof through any mode. A medical practitioner, however, is permitted to make a formal announcement in press regarding the following:

1. On starting practice.
2. On change of type of practice.
3. On changing address.
4. On temporary absence from duty.
5. On resumption of another practice.
6. On succeeding to another practice.
7. Public declaration of charges.

6.1.2 Printing of self photograph, or any such material of publicity in the letter head or on sign board of the consulting room or any such clinical establishment shall be regarded as acts of self advertisement and unethical conduct on the part of the physician. However, printing of sketches, diagrams, picture of human system shall not be treated as unethical.

6.2 Patent and Copyrights: A physician may patent surgical instruments, appliances and medicine or copyright applications, methods and procedures. However, it shall be unethical if the benefits of such patents or copyrights are not made available in situations where the interest of large population is involved.

6.3 Running an Open Shop (Dispensing of Drugs and Appliances by Physicians): A physician should not run an open shop for sale of medicine for dispensing prescriptions prescribed by doctors other than himself or for sale of medical or surgical appliances. It is not unethical for a physician to prescribe or supply drugs, remedies or appliances as long as there is no exploitation of the patient. Drugs prescribed by a physician or brought from the market for a patient should explicitly state the proprietary formulae as well as generic name of the drug.

6.4 Rebates and Commission

6.4.1 A physician shall not give, solicit, or receive nor shall he offer to give solicit or receive, any gift, gratuity, commission or bonus in consideration of or return for the referring, recommending or procuring of any patient for medical, surgical or other treatment. A physician shall not directly or indirectly, participate in or be a party to act of division, transference, assignment, subordination, rebating, splitting or refunding of any fee for medical, surgical or other treatment.

6.4.2 Provisions of para 6.4.1 shall apply with equal force to the referring, recommending or procuring by a physician or any person, specimen or material for diagnostic purposes or other study/work. Nothing in this section, however, shall prohibit payment of salaries by a qualified physician to other duly qualified person rendering medical care under his supervision.

6.5 Secret Remedies: The prescribing or dispensing by a physician of secret remedial agents of which he does not know the composition, or the manufacture or promotion of their use is unethical and as such prohibited. All the drugs prescribed by a physician should always carry a proprietary formula and clear name.

6.6 Human Rights: The physician shall not aid or abet torture nor shall he be a party to either infliction of mental or physical trauma or concealment of torture inflicted by some other person or agency in clear violation of human rights.

6.7 Euthanasia: Practicing euthanasia shall constitute unethical conduct. However, on specific occasion, the question of withdrawing supporting devices to sustain cardiopulmonary function even after brain death, shall be decided only by a team of doctors and not merely by the treating physician alone. A team of doctors shall declare withdrawal of support system. Such team shall consist of the doctor in-charge of the patient, Chief Medical Officer/Medical Officer in-charge of the hospital and a doctor nominated by the in-charge of the hospital from the hospital staff or in accordance with the provisions of the Transplantation of Human Organ Act, 1994.

6.8 **Code of conduct for doctors in their relationship with pharmaceutical and allied health sector industry.**

Action to be taken by the Council for violation of Section 6.8, as amended vide notification dated 10/12/2009, shall be prescribed by further amending the Section 6.8.1 as under:

Section	Action
6.8.1 In dealing with Pharmaceutical and allied health sector industry, a medical practitioner shall follow and adhere to the stipulations given below:	
a. **Gifts:** A medical practitioner shall not receive any gift from any pharmaceutical or allied health-care industry and their sales people or representatives.	**Gifts** more than Rs. 1,000/- up to Rs. 5,000/-: Censure **Gifts** more than Rs. 5,000/- upto Rs. 10,000/-: Removal from Indian Medical Register or State Medical Register for 3 (three) months. **Gifts** more than Rs. 10,000/- to Rs. 50,000/-: Removal from Indian Medical Register or State Medical Register for 6 (six) months.

Section	Action
	Gifts more than Rs. 50,000/- to Rs. 1,00,000/-: Removal from Indian Medical Register or State Medical Register for 1 (one) year. **Gifts** more than Rs. 1,00,000/-: Removal for a period of more than 1 (one) year from Indian Medical Register or State Medical Register.
b. **Travel facilities:** A medical practitioner shall not accept any travel facility inside the country or outside, including rail, road, air, ship, cruise tickets, paid vacations, etc. from any pharmaceutical or allied health-care industry or their representatives for self and family members for vacation or for attending conferences, seminars, workshops, CME program, etc. as a delegate.	**Expenses for travel facilities** more than Rs. 1,000/- up to Rs. 5,000/-: Censure. **Expenses for travel facilities** more than Rs. 5,000/- up to Rs. 10,000/-: Removal from Indian Medical Register or State Medical Register for 3 (three) months. **Expenses for travel facilities** more than Rs. 10,000/- to Rs. 50,000/-: Removal from Indian Medical Register or State medical Register for 6 (six) months. **Expenses for travel facilities** more than more than Rs. 50,000/- to Rs. 1,00,000/-: Removal from Indian Medical Register or State Medical Register for 1 (one) year. **Expenses for travel facilities** more than Rs. 1,00,000/-: Removal for a period of more than 1 (one) year from Indian Medical Register or State Medical Register.
c. **Hospitality:** A medical practitioner shall not accept individually any hospitality like hotel accommodation for self and family members under any pretext.	**Expenses for hospitality** more than Rs. 1,000/- upto Rs. 5,000/-: Censure. **Expenses for hospitality** more than Rs. 5,000/- upto Rs. 10,000/-: Removal from Indian Medical Register or State Medical Register for 3 (three) months. **Expenses for hospitality** more than Rs. 10,000/- to Rs. 50,000/-: Removal from Indian Medical Register or State medical Register for 6 (six) months. **Expenses for hospitality** more than more than Rs. 50,000/- to Rs. 1,00,000/: Removal from Indian Medical Register or State Medical Register for 1 (one) year. **Expenses for hospitality** more than Rs. 1,00,000/-: Removal for a period of more than 1 (one) year from Indian Medical Register or State Medical Register.

Section	Action
d. **Cash or monetary grants:** A medical practitioner shall not receive any cash or monetary grants from any pharmaceutical and allied health-care industry for individual purpose in individual capacity under any pretext. Funding for medical research, study etc. can only be received through approved institutions by modalities laid down by law/rules/guidelines adopted by such approved institutions, in a transparent manner. It shall always be fully disclosed.	**Cash or monetary grants** more than Rs. 1,000/- up to Rs. 5,000/-: Censure **Cash or monetary grants** more than Rs. 5,000/- up to Rs. 10,000/-: Removal from Indian Medical Register or State Medical Register for 3 (three) months. **Cash or monetary grants** more than Rs. 10,000/- to Rs. 50,000/-: Removal from Indian Medical Register or State Medical Register for 6 (six) months. **Cash or monetary grants** more than more than Rs. 50,000/- to Rs. 1,00,000/-: Removal from Indian Medical Register or State Medical Register for 1 (one) year. **Cash or monetary grants** more than Rs. 1,00,000/-: Removal for a period of more than 1 (one) year from Indian Medical Register or State Medical Register.
e. **Medical research:** A medical practitioner may carry out, participate in, work in research projects funded by pharmaceutical and allied healthcare industries. A medical practitioner is obliged to know that the fulfillment of the following items (i) to (vii) will be an imperative for undertaking any research assignment/project funded by industry—for being proper and ethical. Thus, in accepting such a position a medical practitioner shall: i. Ensure that the particular research proposal(s) has the due permission from the competent concerned authorities. ii. Ensure that such a research project(s) has the clearance of national/state/institutional ethics committees/bodies. iii. Ensure that it fulfils all the legal requirements prescribed for medical research. iv. Ensure that the source and amount of funding is publicly disclosed at the beginning itself.	First time censure, and thereafter removal of name from Indian Medical Register or State Medical Register for a period depending upon the violation of the clause.

Section	Action
v. Ensure that proper care and facilities are provided to human volunteers, if they are necessary for the research project(s). vi. Ensure that undue animal experimentations are not done and when these are necessary they are done in a scientific and a humane way. vii. Ensure that while accepting such an assignment a medical practitioner shall have the freedom to publish the results of the research in the greater interest of the society by inserting such a clause in the MoU or any other documents/ agreement for any such assignment.	
f. **Maintaining professional autonomy:** In dealing with pharmaceutical and allied health-care industry a medical practitioner shall always ensure that there shall never be any compromise either with his/her own professional autonomy and/or with the autonomy and freedom of the medical institution.	First time censure, and thereafter removal of name from Indian Medical Register or State Medical Register.
g. **Affiliation:** A medical practitioner may work for pharmaceutical and allied health-care industries in advisory capacities, as consultants, as researchers, as treating doctors or in any other professional capacity. In doing so, a medical practitioner shall always: i. Ensure that his professional integrity and freedom are maintained. ii. Ensure that patients interest are not compromised in any way. iii. Ensure that such affiliations are within the law. iv. Ensure that such affiliations/employments are fully transparent and disclosed.	First time censure, and thereafter removal of name from Indian Medical Register or State Medical Register for a period depending upon the violaton of the clause.

Section	Action
h. **Endorsement:-** A medical racti-tioner shall not endorse any drug or product of the industry publically. Any study conducted on the efficacy or otherwise of such products shall be presented to and/or through appro-priate scientific bodies or published in appropriate scientific journals in a proper way.	First time censure, and thereafter re-moval of name from Indian Medical Register or State Medical Register.

CHAPTER 7

7. MISCONDUCT: The following acts of commission or omission on the part of a physician shall constitute professional misconduct rendering him/her liable for disciplinary action.

7.1 Violation of the Regulations: If he/she commits any violation of these regulations.

7.2 If he/she does not maintain the medical records of his/her indoor patients for a period of three years as per regulation 1.3 and refuses to provide the same within 72 hours when the patient or his/her authorized representative makes a request for it as per the regulation 1.3.2.

7.3 If he/she does not display the registration number accorded to him/her by the State Medical Council or the Medical Council of India in his clinic, prescriptions and certificates, etc., issued by him or violates the provisions of regulation 1.4.2.

7.4 Adultery or Improper Conduct: Abuse of professional position by committing adultery or improper conduct with a patient or by maintaining an improper association with a patient will render a physician liable for disciplinary action as provided under the Indian Medical Council Act, 1956 or the concerned State Medical Council Act.

7.5 Conviction by Court of Law: Conviction by a Court of Law for offences involving moral turpitude/Criminal Acts.

7.6 Sex Determination Tests: On no account sex determination test shall be undertaken with the intent to terminate the life of a female fetus developing in her mother's womb, unless there are other absolute indications for termination of pregnancy as specified in the Medical Termination of Pregnancy Act, 1971. Any act of termination of pregnancy of normal female fetus amounting to female feticide shall be regarded as professional misconduct on the part of the physician leading to penal erasure besides rendering him liable to criminal proceedings as per the provisions of this Act.

7.7 Signing Professional Certificates, Reports and other Documents: Registered medical practitioners are in certain cases bound by law to give, or may from time to time be called upon or requested to give certificates, notification, reports and other documents of similar character signed by them in their professional capacity for subsequent use in the courts or for administrative purposes, etc. Any registered practitioner who is shown to have signed or given under his name and authority any such certificate, notification, report or document of a similar character which is untrue, misleading or improper, is liable to have his name deleted from the register.

7.8 A registered medical practitioner shall not contravene the provisions of the Drugs and Cosmetics Act and regulations made thereunder. Accordingly,

(a) prescribing steroids/psychotropic drugs when there is no absolute medical indication;

(b) selling schedule 'H' & 'L' drugs and poisons to the public except to his patient; in contravention of the above provisions shall constitute gross professional misconduct on the part of the physician.

7.9 Performing or enabling unqualified person to perform an abortion or any illegal operation for which there is no medical, surgical or psychological indication.

7.10 A registered medical practitioner shall not issue certificates of efficiency in modern medicine to unqualified or non-medical person.

(**Note:** The foregoing does not restrict the proper training and instruction of bonafide students, midwives, dispensers, surgical attendants, or skilled mechanical and technical assistants and therapy assistants under the personal supervision of physicians).

7.11 A physician should not contribute to the lay press articles and give interviews regarding diseases and treatments which may have the effect of advertising himself or soliciting practices, but is open to write to the lay press under his own name on matters of public health, hygienic living or to deliver public lectures, give talks on the radio/TV/internet chat for the same purpose and send announcement of the same to lay press.

7.12 An institution run by a physician for a particular purpose such as a maternity home, nursing home, private hospital, rehabilitation center or any type of training institution, etc. may be advertised in the lay press, but such advertisements should not contain anything more than the name of the institution, type of patients admitted, type of training and other facilities offered and the fees.

7.13 It is improper for a physician to use an unusually large sign board and write on it anything other than his name, qualifications obtained from a university or a statutory body, titles and name of his speciality, registration number including the name of the State Medical Council under which registered. The same should be the contents of his prescription papers. It is improper to affix a sign-board on a chemist's shop or in places where he does not reside or work.

7.14 The registered medical practitioner shall not disclose the secrets of a patient that have been learnt in the exercise of his/her profession except:

i. in a couart of law under orders of the Presiding Judge;

ii. in circumstances where there is a serious and identified risk to a specific person and/or community; and
iii. notifiable diseases.

In case of communicable/notifiable diseases, concerned public health authorities should be informed immediately.

7.15 The registered medical practitioner shall not refuse on religious grounds alone to give assistance in or conduct of sterility, birth control, circumcision and medical termination of pregnancy when there is medical indication, unless the medical practitioner feels himself/herself incompetent to do so.

7.16 Before performing an operation the physician should obtain in writing the consent from the husband or wife, parent or guardian in the case of minor, or the patient himself as the case may be. In an operation which may result in sterility the consent of both husband and wife is needed.

7.17 A registered medical practitioner shall not publish photographs or case reports of his/her patients without their permission, in any medical or other journal in a manner by which their identity could be made out. If the identity is not to be disclosed, the consent is not needed.

7.18 In the case of running of a nursing home by a physician and employing assistants to help him/her, the ultimate responsibility rests on the physician.

7.19 A Physician shall not use touts or agents for procuring patients.

7.20 A Physician shall not claim to be specialist unless he has a special qualification in that branch.

7.21 No act of *in vitro* fertilization or artificial insemination shall be undertaken without the informed consent of the female patient and her spouse as well as the donor. Such consent shall be obtained in writing only after the patient is provided, at her own level of comprehension, with sufficient information about the purpose, methods, risks, inconveniences, disappointments of the procedure and possible risks and hazards.

7.22 Research: Clinical drug trials or other research involving patients or volunteers as per the guidelines of ICMR can be undertaken, provided ethical considerations are borne in mind. Violation of existing ICMR guidelines in this regard shall constitute misconduct. Consent taken from the patient for trial of drug or therapy which is not as per the guidelines shall also be construed as misconduct.

CHAPTER 8

8. PUNISHMENT AND DISCIPLINARY ACTION

8.1 It must be clearly understood that the instances of offences and of professional misconduct which are given above do not constitute and are not intended to constitute a complete list of the infamous acts which calls for disciplinary action, and that by issuing this notice the Medical Council of

India and or State Medical Councils are in no way precluded from considering and dealing with any other form of professional misconduct on the part of a registered practitioner. Circumstances may and do arise from time to time in relation to which there may occur questions of professional misconduct which do not come within any of these categories. Every care should be taken that the code is not violated in letter or spirit. In such instances as in all others, the Medical Council of India and/or State Medical Councils have to consider and decide upon the facts brought before the Medical Council of India and/ or State Medical Councils.

8.2 It is made clear that any complaint with regard to professional misconduct can be brought before the appropriate Medical Council for Disciplinary action. Upon receipt of any complaint of professional misconduct, the appropriate Medical Council would hold an enquiry and given opportunity to the registered medical practitioner to be heard in person or by pleader. If the medical practitioner is found to be guilty of committing professional misconduct, the appropriate Medical Council may award such punishment as deemed necessary or may direct the removal altogether or for a specified period, from the register of the name of the delinquent registered practitioner. Deletion from the register shall be widely publicized in local press as well as in the publications of different Medical Associations/Societies/Bodies.

8.3 In case the punishment of removal from the register is for a limited period, the appropriate council may also direct that the name so removed shall be restored in the register after the expiry of the period for which the name was ordered to be removed.

8.4 Decision on complaint against delinquent physician shall be taken within a time limit of 6 months.

8.5 During the pendency of the complaint the appropriate council may restrain the physician from performing the procedure or practice which is under scrutiny.

8.6 Professional incompetence shall be judged by peer group as per guidelines prescribed by Medical Council of India.

8.7 Where either on a request or otherwise the Medical Council of India is informed that any complaint against a delinquent physician has not been decided by a State Medical Council within a period of six months from the date of receipt of complaint by it and further the MCI has reason to believe that there is no justified reason for not deciding the complaint within the said prescribed period, the Medical Council of India may:

i. Impress upon the concerned State Medical Council to conclude and decide the complaint within a time bound schedule;

ii. May decide to withdraw the said complaint pending with the concerned State Medical Council straightaway or after the expiry of the period which had been stipulated by the MCI in accordance with para(i) above, to itself and refer the same to the Ethical Committee of the Council for its expeditious disposal in a period of not more than six months from the receipt of the complaint in the office of the Medical Council of India."

8.8 Any person aggrieved by the decision of the State Medical Council on any complaint against a delinquent physician, shall have the right to file an appeal to the MCI within a period of 60 days from the date of receipt of the order passed by the said Medical Council:

Provided that the MCI may, if it is satisfied that the appellant was prevented by sufficient cause from presenting the appeal within the aforesaid period of 60 days, allow it to be presented within a further period of 60 days.

Index

A

B

C

D

E

F

G

T

U

V

W

Y